Perimenopause—
Preparing for the Change

How to Order:
Single copies may be ordered from Prima Publishing, P.O. Box 1260BK, Rocklin, CA 95677; telephone (916) 632-4400. Quantity discounts are also available. On your letterhead, include information concerning the intended use of the books and the number of books you wish to purchase.

Perimenopause—
Preparing for the Change

A Guide to the Early Stages
of Menopause and Beyond

Nancy Lee Teaff, M.D.
Kim Wright Wiley

Prima Publishing

PRIMA PUBLISHING and colophon are trademarks of Prima Communications, Inc.

Library of Congress Cataloging-in-Publication Data

Teaff, Nancy.
    Perimenopause: preparing for the change / Nancy Teaff, Kim Wright Wiley.
        p.   cm.
    Includes index.
    ISBN 1-55958-579-X
    ISBN 0-7615-0437-0 (pbk.)
    1. Menopause—Popular works. I. Wiley, Kim Wright. II. Title.
RG186.T43 1994
618.1'75—dc20   94-21795
                                  CIP

97 98 99 00 01 AA 10 9 8 7 6 5 4

Printed in the United States of America

To our daughters: Julia, Mary Kate, and Leigh

Contents

5   *Risky Business: Heart Disease,*
    Osteoporosis, and Breast Cancer   77

Foreword

I am pleased to introduce this valuable contribution to women's health literature. As a clinician and observer of the women's health scene I have long noted the need for more education about the changes which occur at midlife. Many patients come to me with questions about menopause and they're coming at younger and younger ages.

In my experience fear of the unknown is always worse than the actual occurence. The authors of *Perimenopause—Preparing for the Change* have addressed the major issues of midlife, including the important physical and emotional changes which occur as the ovaries produce less estrogen. Subjects such as fertility potential, contraception, the risks and benefits of hormone replacement therapy and preventative measures to improve general health are addressed in an enjoyable and readable style.

Menopause is indeed a change and there will be challenges to master and mountains to climb, but it can be weathered with style and grace if you have a good map and don't forget to pack your sense of humor. This book is not only a guide for those about to embark on perimenopause, but also helpful for women who have completed this life stage and need some closure on what may have been a confusing experience. Discovering that one is, after all, merely normal can be quite a relief.

Mary G. Hammond, M.D.
President Elect, American Fertility Society
North Carolina Center for Reproductive Medicine

Preface

Kim's Story

During the writing of this book, it was Nancy's job to be the expert and my job to be the idiot. I'd read something and say, "I didn't know that."

She'd say, "Come on, you're kidding."

"No, really. I never heard that word in my whole life."

"How could you not know that? You're a bright woman." And so went the ping-pong ball of our conversations as we debated what belonged in the book and what didn't.

Before she became a reproductive endocrinologist, Nancy was my obstetrician. Like many patients, I was devoted to my doctor and considered it a bonus that she was a woman about my age, as capable of advising me about where to buy good panty hose for the last trimester as she was about epidurals. Still, when she first approached me with her idea for this book, I was skeptical. I was experienced in medical journalism and thought it would be great to work with Nancy, but I knew next to nothing about menopause. That's what I brought to the partnership: my ignorance. I was the one who kept asking the dumb questions.

I'm an unlikely candidate to coauthor a book on peri-menopause for another reason: not only did I know nothing about the subject, but I would have been happy to keep it that way. At 38, I was relieved to have maneuvered my little canoe through the perilous pass of childbirth and early motherhood. My younger child had just gone off to kinder-garten, and I was more than ready to drift for a while, ignoring the dull roar of the waterfall around the next bend. When Nancy proffered her theory that most women have a bad attitude about the advent of menopause, all I could do was shrug. This was news? Of course they have a bad attitude!

My own family history was less than inspiring. I'd seen my grandmother break a hip, which quickly reduced this bright woman—who knew the Latin name for everything and worked the Sunday crossword in ink—to a frightened, trembling shell of her former self. I'd seen my mother, in the fashion of the day, have a hysterectomy at the age of 29 due to fibroid tumors. Her ovaries were left, so there's no telling exactly when she went through menopause, but around the age of 48 she had a severe depression, during which she lost interest in her former activities, stopped seeing friends, and gave up sleeping altogether. The word *menopause* was never mentioned, but the grim lesson was loud and clear: Growing older is all about losing control.

In the typical fashion of my own day, I carpooled with a group of girlfriends to a Planned Parenthood clinic in order to get on the Pill. I waited until we were all in separate rooms, then sheepishly confessed to the doctor that I was still a virgin. She patted my shoulder, gave me the prescription anyway, and said, "Forewarned is forearmed, honey."

A decade later I married, had a daughter, then a son. No surprises allowed. But on some subconscious level I believed that any control I had over my body existed because I was young, and that when you get older things just happen to you. I knew it was politically incorrect to fear aging, and in truth it wasn't the sags and bags I dreaded but the passivity.

The women I interviewed for this book were a revelation! I did my first interview and thought, "She's great—but she can't be typical." Then the second woman, and the third, turned out to be just as energetic and funny. I spoke with a lot of fascinating 50-year-olds in the course of writing this book, and I hope the women quoted surprise you as much as they surprised me. Every day there are more women out there who are challenging the stereotypes about perimenopause, refusing to be victimized or even slowed down.

In a way, our generation is carpooling to the menopause clinic and it may look like we're getting there a couple of years too early. But if I've learned anything from the interviews, it's that the women who most successfully handle perimenopause are those who meet the condition head-on. These women don't wait until they are unable to function; they respond to the first signs of change and persist even in the face of bewildering symptoms and an often-indifferent medical community. If you want to be able to continue working, traveling, feeling good, having sex, maybe even making babies during the perimenopausal years, preparation is everything. Forewarned is forearmed, honey.

Nancy's Story

I've been seeing menopausal and perimenopausal women for the last 12 years, first as an ob-gyn and now as a reproductive endocrinologist. My first clue that treating menopause wasn't as easy as medical school cracked it up to be came early in my practice when I realized that Premarin, the most commonly prescribed form of estrogen, didn't cure every woman's symptoms. Although their hot flashes were relieved, some women actually felt worse. This led me to explore other estrogen preparations, as well as to learn more about menopause by listening to my patients. Much of my practice involves infertile couples, but as women wait longer and longer to attempt pregnancy, my menopause and infertility endeavors overlap more frequently. Understanding reproduction "from soup to nuts" enables me to apply the most up-to-date information in my treatment of both groups of patients.

As I stood in the shower one morning before work, I thought about what I wished women knew about their health before they came to see me. It seemed as though my menopausal patients were looking to me to fix their lives. I don't have a maternal attitude, and my approach has always been to inform women and let them make their own decisions concerning treatment. It bothered me that they were so behindhand in responding to symptoms that had, in many cases, been evolving for years.

I'm a proactive person, and I wanted to see this quality in my patients as well. I'd read Gail Sheehy's landmark book *The Silent Passage: Menopause* but saw it as more reactive—for the woman who says, "I've stopped my periods and I feel awful, so what do I do now?" The volume and breadth of information I wanted my patients to have would require a book, a daunting thought for a busy practitioner. Then I remembered Kim, for whom I'd provided background material for several articles on women's health. She had written clear reviews of complex topics, and I knew she would bring an eclectic perspective to this subject. Fortunately, I was able to sell her on the idea.

This book has been fun to write. Kim and I have laughed a great deal, particularly at some of the responses we've gotten from other people. When I went to a local bookstore and asked where the books on menopause were, the male employee at the service desk suggested I look in the "Aging" section. His female co-worker directed me to "Women's Health" and added, "I'll get him later." Kim and I have tried to bring some humor to what is an unnerving subject for many baby boomer women. We were never going to get old, right?

I hope that this book encourages women to approach menopause and the years beyond with guts and gusto. If a woman has the right attitude, then, whatever lies ahead, she'll be ready with the best information and best health care she can have. Most of the women I know are way beyond thinking about their "golden years." They're looking for something better. Heck, they're going for platinum!

1

⚜

Perimenopause: Preparing for the Change

We women of the baby boomer generation have had unprecedented control over our reproductive lives. Unlike our mothers and grandmothers, we have been able to decide how many children we will have, when we will have them, and—thanks to the prevalence of Lamaze and other widely taught methods and support systems—to some extent even *how* we will have them. The generation of women currently approaching menopause has come to expect, if not complete control over their medical decisions, at least access to the complete facts.

But even though we have been able to choose so much about our reproductive lives, two aspects remain out of our hands: we cannot predict when it will begin or when it will end. Menarche and menopause are still passages that women enter with fragmentary information. These two landmark events seem to thrust themselves upon us with a timing all their own, leaving us mumbling, "Wait, I'm not ready."

While we can't control the when of menopause, we will, because of our sheer numbers, be able to control the how. Within the next decade, 21 million women will enter menopause, which guarantees that when the baby boomers "go through the change," it will be a media event, the Next Big Thing. In 1900, fewer than 5 million women in this country were older than 50. By the end of the 1990s, more than 50 million American women will be over 50, making us the largest group of women ever to hit menopause, as well as the most vocal.

The prototype of the menopausal woman is changing drastically. A 50-year-old American woman today is statistically likely to be working, may have young children still in the home, and, more than any previous generation, is responsible for the care of her own aging parents. The image of the granny rocking on the porch is ludicrously outdated, and the standard advice given menopausal women 30 years ago—"Just lie down until you feel better"—simply doesn't work for a woman with a full-time job, a five-year-old child, and a mother living in her guest room. "I can't have downtime," says a 48-year-old surgical nurse with three teenagers. "I can't even afford a down week."

Not only will we be going through the change in astounding numbers, but our generation will be menopausal for decades. If you menstruate from age 12 to age 49 and live to be 80 (the average life expectancy for women born in the 1950s), you'll spend half of your adult life in menopause. When you consider how much time and energy we've devoted to preparing ourselves for relatively transient physical passages, such as pregnancy, it clearly behooves us to learn as much as possible about menopause.

What Is Perimenopause?

Perimenopause means the years surrounding menopause (*peri* as in *perimeter*). Perimenopause is best defined as the transition between the time you begin to experience menopausal symptoms, usually the mid- to late 40s, and the time when your periods actually stop, the average age being 51. Some women develop symptoms in their 30s, so perimenopause can last as long as 15 years, but a more typical length is six years.

The term *perimenopause* has entered our vocabulary because of an increasing awareness that menopause is not an event, it's a process. The ovaries begin producing less consistent levels of estrogen when a woman is in her 30s, and by her mid-40s she may be experiencing signs of estrogen withdrawal, such as hot flashes or mood swings, even though actual menopause is still a decade away. Since many woman define menopause as the point when their periods stop, a woman enduring early symptoms probably will not link them to hormonal changes. She's apt to dismiss her irritability or memory lapses as the result of stress, aging, or a case of "PMS from hell."

Even if she does become concerned enough to visit her doctor, she may well be told she's too young to be in menopause. Some physicians are more alert to perimenopausal symptoms than others, but many maintain that you're either "in" menopause or you aren't—and if you're still having periods, lady, you aren't "in" anything, no matter how many hot flashes you've had. Given that not all members of the medical community are experts on this issue, it's wise to take perimenopause into your own hands by being well-informed, sensitive to changes in your body, and willing to search for a physician who is on the same wavelength.

When Will Menopause Occur?

Although it would be reassuring to think you could sit down with a calculator, add and subtract all the individual factors, hit the total button, and say, "Aha, I'll enter menopause at 48," the truth is that it's extremely difficult to predict when menopause will begin for an individual woman. Certain natural variables, such as race or body type, affect when you'll go through menopause, as do lifestyle variables such as the age at which you had your first child, past illnesses or surgeries, and whether or not you smoke.

There's a common misconception that women who begin their periods earlier than average will enter menopause earlier than average, and, conversely, that women who didn't begin having periods until they were 14 or 15 will be well into their 50s before they experience menopause. This is a tempting theory to accept, both because it makes the onset of menopause easier to predict and because it only seems fair to assume that the first people to board the reproductive school bus in the morning would be the first ones to get off in the afternoon. Alas, the route is nowhere near so regular. Research shows no correlation between the age of menarche and the age of menopause.

Another old theory holds more water: the odds are you'll enter menopause at about the same age as your mother. Unfortunately, since hysterectomies were common in our mothers' generation, the age at which your mother would have naturally experienced menopause may be something you'll never know.

Numerous other factors must be tallied—some of them logical and some seemingly random and bizarre. The average age of menopause is 51. Start with that figure, and then consider these findings:

♦ Thinner, smaller-boned women go through menopause earlier than heavy or big-boned women.

♦ Women who have never had children go through menopause earlier than women who have borne several. In fact, research indicates that each child you bear will delay the onset of menopause by about five months.

♦ White women go through menopause earlier than black women.

- Smokers go through menopause earlier than non-smokers.

- Women who live at higher altitudes go through menopause sooner than women who live at sea level.

- Illness can delay the onset of menopause, especially cancer of the breast or uterus, fibroids in the uterus, or diabetes.

- Women who have suffered from poor nutrition throughout their lives will go through menopause earlier.

- Somewhat conversely, a higher standard of living is associated with an earlier menopause.

- A hysterectomy or tubal ligation can bring an earlier menopause, as can a history of several abortions. Note: If the ovaries are removed in a hysterectomy, menopause is immediate, but even if the ovaries are not removed, the removal of the uterus appears to cause the woman to enter menopause a few years earlier than she would have normally.

- If you had shorter than average menstrual cycles, i.e., fewer than 25 days, you are more likely to experience menopause earlier.

- If you had your first child after the age of 40, menopause will be later than average.

- Women who have been on birth control pills for many years often experience a slightly later menopause. Note: This can be confusing because oral contraceptives may provide enough estrogen to keep your periods coming, even after menopause has begun. In the absence of the most obvious symptom, skipped periods, a woman on birth control pills may enter menopause without realizing it.

Any factor that has affected a woman's reproductive history could potentially modify the age at which she'll go through menopause. You and your sister may have begun life with similar genetic blueprints, but if the choices each of you subsequently made about contraception and child-bearing override your inborn similarities, she may enter menopause five years earlier or five years later than you.

We have heard a male doctor, speaking before a group of women at a seminar on PMS, rather offensively claim that the women of our generation have "tinkered with their reproductive capabilities." The women in the audience argued that contraception, abortion, or a decision to delay childbearing hardly qualify as "tinkering," and we agree. But it is true that the track record of our female relatives won't tell the whole story for us. For starters, we have borne fewer children and thus had more menstrual cycles than any previous generation. And if you consider that for centuries women married shortly after puberty and remained either pregnant or nursing for most of their fertile lives, it's clear that the average woman living today has many more periods than a woman living 500 years ago experienced. In fact, today's woman probably has quite a few more periods than her own grandmother had. Will the number of menstrual cycles a woman has in her lifetime ultimately affect when or how she enters menopause? No one knows yet, but such questions only throw more variables into the pot.

The best approach is to be aware of the influencing factors, but not overly dependent upon them for guidance. Familiarize yourself with the harbingers of perimenopause, so that you will recognize them whenever they appear. After all, the bottom line is you don't go through menopause when the charts say you'll go through it. You go through it when you go through it.

Medically Induced Menopause

Not every woman enters menopause gradually. If your ovaries are removed surgically or you undergo radiation or chemotherapy treatments intense enough to halt ovarian function, your menopause will be immediate. A medically induced menopause is tough for three reasons. First, your estrogen withdrawal is more abrupt than the usual winding-down process of perimenopause, so your symptoms are likely to be more dramatic as well. It's like driving a car at 60 miles per hour and suddenly slamming on the brakes. Secondly, you are already under tremendous stress due to the hysterectomy or cancer, and the unexpected addition of a whole new set of problems may seem like too much to bear. Finally, our society offers virtually no support or recognition for the 31-year-old in menopause. If she's grieving over the loss of her ability to bear children or worrying about how this is going to affect her sexuality through the years, she may have no one to whom she can talk.

More than one-third of the women in the U.S. have hysterectomies. When an oophorectomy (removal of the ovaries) is part of the procedure, some women report that the hot flashes of menopause begin within days after the surgery.

It is vital for women experiencing medically induced menopause to find an empathetic doctor, one who not only can help them through the rough transition, but who is also aware of the long-term health implications of their condition. A woman going through an early menopause will be in estrogen depletion perhaps decades longer than the average woman, and since estrogen protects the heart and bones, she and her doctor will need to devise a program to counteract the loss.

Women in early menopause might also consider talking to a therapist or joining a support group. The standard comfort for most women in menopause is that everyone they know is going through it too. Lacking that consolation, you'll need to search harder to find women in the same boat. Many hospitals have support groups for women recovering from cancer, and larger hospitals tend to divide the groups by age or type of illness. By talking to one another, you can share information about doctors, treatments, and coping strategies while assuaging the loneliness that often accompanies an "out of season" menopause.

The Life Cycle of the Ovary

Menopause may culminate in the uterus, but it begins in the ovary.

Six months without periods (amenorrhea) is the most recognized clinical definition of menopause, which means that the symptom by which we diagnose menopause is actually one of the last steps in the process. The sometimes abrupt cessation of menstruation led to the euphemism "the change," as if a woman awakes one morning to find herself menopausal. But this obvious symptom was preceded by many less noticeable pauses in ovarian function, and an overemphasis on skipped periods is one reason perimenopause is so often ignored.

The Egg Count

We contend that menopause is a process that begins before you're aware of it, but would you believe it starts before birth? In some ways, the blueprint for a woman's menopause is established while she's an embryo, for by the time a female fetus reaches 20 weeks of gestation, her ovaries have a fixed number of follicles containing eggs. The number of eggs drops throughout the pregnancy from a high of 2 million to the approximately 700,000 viable eggs a baby girl has at birth.

As the child grows, the eggs contained in her ovarian follicles continue to die. By puberty she has approximately 400,000 left, still a staggering number, but because only one follicle of a stimulated group of follicles will mature and release an egg, the young woman can expect to experience "only" about 500 ovulations in her lifetime.

By the time menopause approaches, the ovaries have begun to run out of the follicles that respond to the follicle-stimulating hormone (also known as FSH) which prepares the follicles for egg release. FSH causes one follicle to grow and the ovum within it to mature. The layer of cells within the follicle secrete estradiol, the body's natural form of estrogen, which in turn causes the uterine lining to thicken in anticipation of receiving a fertilized egg. The stage of the menstrual cycle that precedes ovulation is the follicular phase; if the follicles that contain the egg are not stimulated by FSH, or if they aren't capable of responding to the FSH, no estrogen is produced. Without estrogen, the uterine lining doesn't thicken, and there is nothing to slough off as a period.

An FSH measurement higher than 40 anytime from the second through the sixth day of the menstrual cycle is considered a reliable indicator that menopause has occurred. It's a bit confusing: a high measurement of FSH indicates menopause is approaching, and a low measurement means the ovaries are still functioning. This seeming paradox is tribute to how hard the human reproductive system strives to keep going. As menopause nears, FSH surges in a last-ditch effort to force the follicles to release eggs—and estrogen. If you suspect menopause is approaching, you should ask your physician for a FSH test, because a high FSH reading can signal perimenopause more accurately than skipped periods. The testing procedure is discussed later in this chapter.

As production of estrogen, and the post-ovulation hormone, progesterone, begins to taper off, the menstrual cycle will change. Cycle length may decrease. A woman used to a 28-day cycle may find herself menstruating every 25 days. A previously regular woman may skip a period altogether.

Shorter cycles are one clue that a woman may no longer be ovulating. Ovulation is generally considered the midpoint of a menstrual cycle. As estrogen production decreases, the number of days before the cycle midpoint will decrease. As progesterone decreases, the number of days after the cycle midpoint will vary. Obviously, if both hormones are absent or present only in small amounts, the menstrual cycle will alter to a marked degree (see Figure 1.1).

The menstrual changes women experience in perimenopause can take many forms—heavier periods, lighter periods, skipped periods, the sudden advent of PMS or cramps—but they are the first sign that the process is under way.

How Do You Know If You're in Perimenopause?

Besides skipped periods or shorter menstrual cycles, several other symptoms indicate perimenopause. Most common are hot flashes, followed by insomnia, mood swings, loss of concentration or memory, and, finally, vaginal dryness.

Perimenopausal symptoms and suggested courses of treatment are discussed in detail in chapter 3, and the run-through here is only to help you in self-diagnosis of the earliest stages. If you have several of these symptoms, consider calling your doctor to schedule FSH and estradiol/estrogen tests.

♦ Hot flashes and night sweats
♦ Interrupted sleep or insomnia
♦ Irritability
♦ Anxiety
♦ Loss of concentration
♦ Headaches (especially premenstrual migraines)
♦ Vaginal dryness
♦ Less interest in sex *(continued on page 12)*

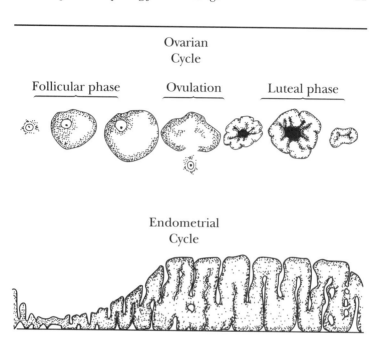

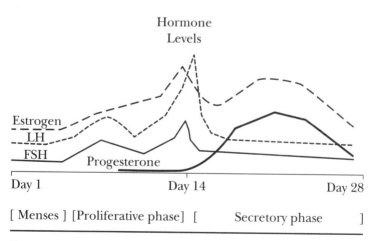

Figure 1.1 Sequence of events in a normal menstrual cycle showing the relationship of hormone levels to the events in the ovary and the uterus.

♦ Urinary stress incontinence

♦ Mood swings

Obviously, many of these symptoms are interconnected. If you have such severe night sweats that you develop insomnia, your concentration will suffer and you'll be too tired for sex. From there the dominoes just keep falling, and what begins as a physical problem can escalate into a psychological problem. The mood swings may make you feel as though you're back in seventh grade, and indeed the hormonal changes of perimenopause are more like those of puberty than you might guess.

Reverse Puberty

In puberty, early estrogen production leads to breast development and the growth of the endometrium (uterine lining), which will ultimately shed itself and become the girl's first menstrual cycle. During the first year or two of menarche, cycles are often irregular and usually not ovulatory. Estrogen production is also erratic, and these fluctuating hormonal levels, coupled with the daily traumas of adolescent life, lead to the wild mood swings that are so much a part of being a pubescent girl.

In menopause, the reverse happens, with similar results. The ovaries are gearing down instead of gearing up, but the dueling hormonal levels can bring on the same mood swings experienced 40 years earlier—and the same helpless feeling that makes a woman wonder, "What's happening to me?"

The key is that a consistent hormonal cycle enables a woman to predict her ups and downs. She may have PMS, but at least she knows when to expect it and can recognize it for what it is. But when the cycle's regularity is destroyed and hormone levels rise and fall in an unpredictable pattern throughout this new non-cycle, the woman may begin to suffer bouts of irritability and depression.

Diagnostic Tests

The two most important diagnostic tests for perimenopause are the follicle-stimulating hormone test and the estrogen (or estradiol) test.

A changing menstrual pattern or hot flashes indicates that your estrogen level is dropping and an FSH test should be done. The test is relatively simple: blood is drawn sometime during the first four to six days of your menstrual cycle (or anytime if you're amenorrhic) for two successive months. If your FSH levels exceed 40 international units on both occasions, the ovary has shut down,

---

Is This PMS or Perimenopause?

Many of the symptoms of perimenopause are also symptoms of PMS, so it's easy to dismiss your complaints as PMS, especially if you're still having regular periods. But you should suspect perimenopause if:

1. You have never had PMS, but now you suddenly do.
2. You always had PMS but a new symptom has kicked in, such as night sweats or headaches.
3. The symptoms don't disappear when your period starts, or soon thereafter.

PMS has cyclic, somewhat predictable patterns of symptoms, while perimenopausal symptoms are less consistent. In perimenopause, you may feel irritable and suffer from insomnia for several months and then the problems abate, only to return six months later. Chart your mood swings in relation to your menstrual cycles. If no pattern emerges and what you seem to be having is monthlong PMS, it may actually be perimenopause.

and you're menopausal. A reading of more than 20 on two separate occasions is enough to suggest you're perimenopausal.

Your estrogen level affects how you feel, making the estrogen test another vital piece of the perimenopausal puzzle. For this test, blood is drawn on day two, three, or four of the menstrual cycle. A low level of estrogen is the most common cause of hot flashes, insomnia, mood swings, vaginal dryness, and the other complaints associated with perimenopause. (Strangely enough, an inappropriately high level of estrogen during days two through four *also* indicates the erratic ovarian function typical of perimenopause. Any deviation from the normal pattern is noteworthy.)

An estrogen check alone suffices for many women, although your physician may opt for a total ovarian hormonal profile. Your testosterone level can be checked anytime, and a low reading is often behind a loss of libido. If you are trying to conceive or having severe problems with menstrual irregularity, your progesterone should be checked after ovulation is thought to have occurred, usually around days 20 to 22 of your menstrual cycle.

An Overall Health Evaluation

Other tests your doctor may suggest are only indirectly related to menopause. This is the time of life when you should begin having regular mammograms and cholesterol checks, if you aren't already. In addition, one of the biggest health challenges faced by older women is osteoporosis, and your risk can be determined through a Dual Energy X-Ray Absorptiometry (DEXA), which measures your current bone mineral content. Much as an early mammogram establishes a baseline against which future screening tests are measured, an early DEXA will help your physician ascertain whether you're losing, maintaining, or building bone mass in the years to come.

Perimenopause is an excellent time to do an overall health evaluation (see Figure 1.2). Your body is telling you that it's changing, and you may want to reassess how you're living with regard to nutrition, exercise, and stress. The point of this advice is not to make you feel fragile, or to suggest that you should run to your doctor with the first symptom, but rather to encourage you to take a proactive stance toward the next 40 years of your life. And if your physican says that you're "too young" to be worrying about such matters, step one should be to look for a new physician.

Your Medical History

Your doctor should begin by asking if you have a personal or family history of:

♦ Heart disease

♦ Liver disease

♦ Cancer—especially whether you or a close female relative has had cancer of the breast, uterus, or ovary

♦ Osteoporosis

♦ Diabetes

Do you have any drug allergies? What medications, if any, are you currently taking?

What about your gynecological history? Take the time to discuss your:

♦ Menstrual patterns

♦ Pregnancy history

♦ Gynecological operations

♦ Any present symptoms of perimenopause

How healthy is your present lifestyle?

♦ Do you smoke? *(continued on page 18)*

Test	30–39 years	40–49 years	50–59 years
1. complete examination	every 4 years	every 4 years	every 4 years
2. blood pressure	every other year	every other year	every other year
3. breast examination	every other year	every year	every year
4. Pap smear	every other year	every other year	every other year
5. pelvic examination	every other year	evey year	every year
6. mammogram	age 36	every other year	every year
7. cholesterol check	every 5 years	every 5 years	every 5 years
8. stool examination	every other year	every other year	every year
9. sigmoidoscopy	–	–	every 4 years
10. electrocardiogram	age 37	age 45	–
11. dental cleaning	twice a year	twice a year	twice a year
12. eye examination	–	–	every 3 years
13. counseling	every year	every year	every year

Figure 1.2 Routine Healthcare Checklist

1. This should include a total medical history of you and your family, lifestyle, and habits.

2. Continuing blood pressure checks are essential since hypertension is the most treatable cause of strokes and is an important factor in heart disease.

3. This should not replace monthly self-exams.

4. For the first three years after sexual activity occurs, Pap smears should be conducted. Provided that these findings are normal, future Pap smears depend upon sexual activity and smoking.

5. Pelvic exams should be conducted along with Pap smears.

6. Mammograms should follow breast exams by your doctor.

7. Cholesterol checks are very important in predicting heart disease.

8. This is important to check for colorectal cancer.

9. This procedure is done in the office and is an inspection of the last 10 to 12 inches of the large intestine.

10. Should have baseline in the late 30s.

11. Cleaning is needed twice a year with check for oral cancer.

12. Exam should include glaucoma screening.

13. Discuss any questions, concerns, risks, lifestyle choices, etc. with your health-care professional.

Figure 1.2 *continued*

♦ Do you exercise on a regular basis?

♦ Do you watch your diet, especially in terms of getting adequate fiber and calcium and limiting your fat intake?

♦ Are you overweight?

A thorough doctor will also take the time to utilize the most important instrument in modern medicine, the chair. You should schedule a conference both to discuss test results and to bring up symptoms or concerns that don't fit into a previously analyzed category — a loss of energy perhaps, or any personal problems that affect your stress level or overall health.

It's vital to assess your personal risk for the "big three": heart disease, osteoporosis, and breast cancer. Use the lists in chapter 5 to make an evaluation. Several listed factors predisposing you toward a certain illness may warrant more frequent screenings than the routinely recom- mended number, as well as more aggressive preventive care. Obviously, not every factor carries equal weight. A family history of breast cancer, for example, is a greater cause for concern than merely being Caucasian. But the lists will help to make you aware of where you are poten- tially at risk.

Why Should You Care?

Why should we become hypersensitive about the approach of menopause? A quick scan of the symptoms may con- vince you that you suffer from all of them—and have, frankly, since birth. You may feel so burdened by the sheer weight of the issues surrounding menopause that you're tempted to say, "I'll just get through it, whenever it comes. Everybody does, including my own mother, who probably never even uttered the word aloud."

The main reason to arm yourself with knowledge now is so you can take a proactive stance. As we've seen, by the time symptoms appear, changes have been going on for months or years beneath the surface. And by the time symptoms become disruptive, you will have missed several opportunities to intervene.

From 15 to 20 percent of women going through menopause report symptoms severe enough to hamper their ability to function at home or at work, while 65 to 80 percent report noticeable symptoms beyond skipped periods. Granted, these complaints are rarely crippling, but why suffer any more than you have to? Going to the doctor only when your symptoms become unbearable is simply not good preventive medicine and certainly not a smart choice for a woman who needs to function at peak ability every day of the month.

Consider the fact that you'll likely be menopausal for decades and ask yourself whether you really want to tough it out for 40 years. If you enter perimenopause with no information and no plans to help yourself through it, you'll undoubtedly survive, but how good are you going to feel? For women of our generation, how well we prepare for menopause may be the ultimate quality-of-life issue.

2

Fertility and Infertility

Call it Murphy's Law of Perimenopause: the women who want to get pregnant, can't, and those who don't want to get pregnant, do. The cruel irony is that the number of 40-something women thronging the infertility clinics is exceeded only by the number of 40-something women thronging the abortion clinics.

Surprisingly, women in their 40s have the second-highest rate of unplanned pregnancy of any age group. Only teenage girls goof more often than we do—and only teenage girls have more abortions. In fact, among women 40 and older, an unplanned pregnancy is more likely to end in abortion than birth; the average is 514 abortions per 1,000 pregnancies.

Why do mature women get pregnant so often by mistake? It's obviously not because they were carried away on a tide of passion in the backseat of a car, but more likely because they didn't realize they were still fertile. Women commonly misinterpret skipped periods for the absence of ovulation, or fail to realize that during perimenopause a woman can produce a nonviable egg in one cycle and a viable egg in the next, essentially rotating between fertility and infertility.

To be absolutely safe, most doctors recommend maintaining contraception for a full year after your last menstrual cycle. This may sound like paranoia, but it's actually self-protective. The challenges of menopause are great enough without adding a surprise pregnancy to the mix.

How to Tell Whether You're Ovulating

As we discussed in chapter 1, the reproductive cycle is not a roulette wheel that is stopped in midspin by the hand of fate. Egg production winds down slowly.

Although men produce sperm throughout their lives, a woman is born with all the eggs she'll ever have. The eggs die off at the rate of about 1,000 per month, but since we begin life with as many as 700,000 eggs, the perimenopausal woman still has about 10,000 eggs left, technically more than enough. As we near menopause, however, the follicle may fail to release an egg each month. Even if released, the egg itself is now more than 40 years old and may no longer be viable, that is, capable of being fertilized and attaching itself to the uterine wall. A woman in her 40s may be popping a nonviable egg three or four cycles per year, which is bad news for the perimenopausal woman who is trying to conceive.

The equally bad news if you're trying *not* to get pregnant is that this same theoretical woman is producing viable eggs during the other months of the year. Natural menopause has occurred in only 11 percent of women aged 45 to 49, so unless she's had surgical intervention, a woman in her late 40s should assume that she is still capable of conceiving.

If you have doubts about whether you're fertile, an FSH test will give you more to go on. The follicle stimulating hormone is actually produced far away from the ovaries, in the pituitary gland at the base of the brain. A normally functioning ovary secretes substances that suppress FSH, and a fertile woman who is still years away from menopause will produce FSH levels of less than 20 mIU/ml (milli international units/milliliter) on cycle days two to six. But as ovarian secretions decline and FSH levels rise, a menopausal woman will produce FSH levels of 40 mIU/ml or higher. A reading between 20 and 40 indicates perimenopause, sporadic ovulation—and the need for continued contraception.

How to Get Pregnant

Over the last 20 years, the number of women older than 35 who are giving birth for the first time has increased dramatically. The tendency to marry later and delay childbearing has resulted in many more 35- to 45-year-old women who are trying either to start a family or to increase their family size as perimenopause approaches.

Clinically, infertility is defined as the inability to conceive within one year. The standard advice is if you've gone a year with unprotected sex and still aren't pregnant, there's a 90 percent chance that something is wrong and you should seek medical advice.

A woman over age 35, however, can't afford to wait a full year before seeking help. There are numerous infertility treatments in use today, but many of them take time. As soon as she decides she wants a baby, a woman over 35 should begin using ovulation predictor kits or basal body temperature (BBT) charting, and if six months of unprotected intercourse don't result in a pregnancy, she should schedule an infertility workup.

The time factor plays out as follows: the risk of infertility rises from 6 percent for women between ages 20 to 24 to 64 percent for women between 40 and 44. Put another way, within 10 months of trying, 80 percent of women under 34 will get pregnant on their own. (Well, they will need a man, or at least sperm.) But only 40 percent of women over 40 conceive within 10 months without any sort of medical intervention.

This doesn't mean that if you're in your 40s you aren't fertile. The chances of your having a baby eventually are still good. The key word is *eventually*. It's your rate of fecundity—the chance of conception during a single menstrual cycle—that falls so sharply in your 40s. There are several reasons:

1. First and foremost, couples in their 40s tend to have sex less frequently than couples in their 20s. You gotta play to win.

2. An egg may not be released every cycle, or a released egg may not be of sufficient quality to be fertilized.

3. Inadequate progesterone production may result in a deficient preparation of the endometrium. If the uterine lining isn't ready, the fertilized egg can't embed itself, and thus no pregnancy ensues. This condition is sometimes referred to as luteal phase deficiency.

4. Endometriosis is common among women in their 40s. Normally, the endometrium either receives the fertilized egg and provides nourishment for an embryo, or, if no fertilization has taken place, is shed as the period. In endometrosis, the uterine lining leaks out through the fallopian tubes and into the pelvic cavity. It can then adhere to the ovaries and to the outside of the uterus, not only preventing conception, but also causing extreme discomfort.

5. Tubal infertility (damaged fallopian tubes) is another potential problem. If the problem is mini-

mal, such as slight scarring, laparoscopic surgery can be done on an outpatient basis. If the damage is more severe, in vitro fertilization (IVF) becomes the treatment of choice, as it bypasses the fallopian tubes altogether.

A reduction in fecundity doesn't occur only in women. Only one-third of males over the age of 40 manage to impregnate their partners within six months. While many of the causes of male infertility, such as undescended testicles or diseases such as mumps, have been present since childhood, environmental factors can also be responsible; a man who previously fathered a child may find himself entering middle age with a reduced sperm count.

An Infertility Workup: What to Expect

A typical fertility workup begins with both partners giving their complete physical—including sexual—histories. Standard tests include a semen analysis for the man, a hormone evaluation for the woman, and a postcoital test to study the interaction between the man's sperm and the woman's cervical mucus. A hysterosalpingrapm (HSG) sounds dreadful but is actually a relatively simple X-ray procedure during which dye is injected into the uterus to see whether it flows through the fallopian tubes, indicating whether they are blocked.

If the woman is approaching 40, the physician may also schedule a laparoscopy as part of the initial workup. Ordinarily a laparoscopy, which allows direct observation of the uterus and fallopian tubes through a small incision made below the navel, is delayed until an HSG indicates an abnormality. But since the HSG cannot detect all problems and even the slightest degree of endometriosis or scar tissue can interfere with an already tenuous fertility, a doctor is likely to schedule a laparoscopy earlier for an older woman.

Infertility Treatments

The method of treatment, of course, depends on the reason for the infertility. If a lack of sperm is the problem, donor insemination will be advised, and the success rate for women over 35 is high: 54 percent conceive over the span of 12 cycles. Blocked fallopian tubes or endometriosis can often be corrected through laparoscopic surgery.

If your hormonal evaluation indicates that the ovary is not functioning, however, prepare yourself for a more lengthy and invasive treatment. As age becomes a factor, a treatment is evaluated not only in terms of how successfully it works but also how quickly it works. Given the catch-22 of perimenopausal fertility—it takes more time to get pregnant and you have less time—in vitro fertilization and similar procedures are often recommended because they have the highest per-cycle likelihood of producing a pregnancy. IVF using donated eggs, for example, has a better than 40 percent percent success rate per cycle.

If your FSH is higher than 25, your estradiol level is over 60 on cycle day three, or you are older than 42, the chances of success using your own eggs is remote. Now is the time to reconsider exactly why you want a child: Are you seeking to reproduce yourself genetically? Do you want the experiences of pregnancy and birth? Or do you simply long to be a parent and the method by which you receive the child is incidental? If your primary objective is parenthood and not necessarily pregnancy, a wider range of options, such as adoption, should be considered. But if you strongly desire the birth experience, then it's literally back to the lab for you.

High-tech Pregnancies

An increasingly common form of assisted pregnancy is in vitro fertilization, popularly known as a "test tube baby."

Either the woman's own egg or a donor's egg is removed from a ripe follicle and fertilized by a sperm cell outside her body. The fertilized egg is allowed to grow and divide for several days before it is inserted into the woman's uterus.

A similar procedure is gamete intra-fallopian transfer, or GIFT. Immediately before ovulation, an egg is removed from either the prospective mother or a donor and then mixed with either her partner's or donor sperm. The sperm-egg mixture is then transferred into the fallopian tubes where fertilization may take place "naturally" inside the mother's body.

Zygote intra-fallopian transfer, or ZIFT, involves the insertion of a zygote (an embryo in its earliest stage) directly into the fallopian tube via laparoscopy. (This zygote is a result of fertilization outside the body in a petri dish.) The zygote moves down the fallopian tube, attaches itself to the uterine wall, and the pregnancy proceeds.

From a layperson's point of view, the three options are not very different. The choice of procedures depends primarily on the program or clinic you're using, whether you have any religious convictions that fertilization must take place inside the body, and your own anatomy. The woman must have functional fallopian tubes for GIFT or ZIFT to work; if your tubes are blocked or damaged, IVF is your best option.

Depending upon the condition of your eggs and your partner's sperm, there are four ways to make a high-tech baby:

1. *Your egg and your partner's sperm.*
   If you have viable eggs and your partner has adequate sperm, the resulting baby will be a genetic mix of the two of you, albeit mixed in a slightly unusual container.

2. *Your eggs and donor sperm.*
   For women with viable eggs who either have no

partner or a partner with inadequate sperm, donor sperm can be used. A variation on artificial insemination, IVF is an option for the woman who is pushing either the age or estrogen limit but still has some healthy eggs left, or whose fallopian tubes are damaged.

3. *Donor eggs and your husband's sperm.*
   If your ovary is faltering, but your partner has viable sperm, you can use a donor egg. As we've seen, the uterus soldiers on for several years after the ovary has retired, so pregnancy is possible even for a woman who is menopausal.

4. *Donor eggs and donor sperm.*
   Even if your eggs and your husband's sperm are both nonviable, you can still have the pregnancy and birth experience.

If you are exhibiting signs of perimenopause but want to have a child, you probably cannot simply let nature take its course. We often speak of people as being either fertile or infertile, but there is a third category between the two, "subfertile," and many perimenopausal women fall into it. If you wait too long to seek medical help, you may end up requiring more invasive and complex treatment than if you had gone in earlier. The payoff in reacting quickly to signs of subfertility is that you have more options, more time, and thus a greater chance of having a baby.

Note: All this talk about "partners" and "husbands" is a matter of linguistic convenience and is not meant to disparage the attempts of single women to achieve motherhood. The obvious truth is that you don't need a husband or even a male partner to become pregnant. You only need sperm, and they're not hard to obtain.

The basic question for a single woman is the same as for her married counterpart: Are your eggs viable? If they are, you can seek pregnancy through artificial insemination. If not, you'll require both donor sperm and eggs, and will need to investigate IVF, GIFT, or ZIFT.

How to Stay Pregnant

Once the fertilized egg attaches itself to the uterine wall, the perimenopausal mother faces another hurdle. The risk of spontaneous abortion, or miscarriage, increases significantly as a woman ages. A 30-year-old woman has a 10 percent chance of miscarriage, rising to a 33 percent risk for women aged 40 to 44; a woman over the age of 45 is more likely to miscarry than to bring a pregnancy to term. FSH can also be a barometer of how prone you are to miscarry: a high FSH level at any age portends a greater likelihood of miscarriage.

Furthermore, babies born to older mothers bear a well-publicized risk of chromosomal abnormalities. Amniocentesis and chorionic villus sampling (CVS)—tests that screen for a variety of defects—are recommended for women who will be 35 or older when they give birth. CVS diagnoses a range of genetic abnormalities and can be done as early as the 10th week of pregnancy, which means it can give you great peace of mind. Amniocentesis involves withdrawal of fluid from the amniotic sac, and because it is performed rather late in a pregnancy (around the 16th week), is done less routinely to screen for genetic disorders.

If a woman over 40 begins her pregnancy without a high-risk factor working against her, has the early screening tests, and does not miscarry, she will likely deliver a healthy baby. The horror stories about older mothers are often linked to preexisting medical conditions such as diabetes, hypertension, and obesity, or a family history of genetic abnormalities. A healthy 40-year-old with adequate prenatal care can expect a positive outcome.

How Not to Get Pregnant

Of course, if you don't want to have a baby, all of the statistics in the previous sections can be inverted. A woman in her late 30s who is using no contraception has a 30 to 50 percent chance of conceiving, so this is no time to get sloppy about birth control. The estrogen in hormone replacement therapy (HRT) may actually increase ovarian function, and consequently increase the chances of conception.

Sterilization of one member of a couple is the most common way of preventing unwanted pregnancy in the United States; about one-half of married couples choose this method. In terms of reversible contraception, oral contraceptives are most popular, with 20 percent of women aged 18 to 44 using the Pill.

Using oral contraceptives has an added advantage because the Pill contains sufficient quantities of estrogen and progesterone to help control hot flashes and irregular periods, two of the most common complaints of perimenopause. Oral contraceptives in effect serve as hormone replacement therapy, promoting the maintenance of bone density and regular menstrual cycles. A growing number of women opt to take the Pill throughout their 40s and then switch directly to HRT when they become menopausal.

Unless a woman smokes or has another high-risk factor, such as blood clots or previous cardiovascular disease, the benefits to remaining on oral contraceptives outweigh the risks. The Pill is safer than pregnancy, especially for women in their 40s, and women approaching perimenopause can often use the lowest dosage since their ovarian function is already lessened and thus easier to suppress.

The Pill is followed in frequency of use by condoms, the rhythm method, coitus interruptus, diaphragms, IUDs, and spermicide. (Other methods that became available only recently include the Depo-Provera injection, the Norplant implant, and the female condom.) It may surprise you to learn that the clumsy attempts at contraception of the teenage years—withdrawal and the rhythm method—reappear among couples in their 40s.

Obviously, withdrawal and attempting to have intercourse during the supposedly safe times have always been risky, and become more so when the woman is having irregular menstrual cycles. The high failure rate of these methods is reflected in the abortion statistics for women in our age group.

If you have multiple partners or your partner has multiple partners, condoms are a must, as they reduce your exposure to venereal diseases, including AIDS. The female condom is especially effective because more of the vulva and the base of the penis are protected, thus lessening the chance of contracting herpes or genital warts. It's noteworthy that women who use diaphragms have one-third the risk of cervical cancer of women who use no such protection, possibly due to the antiviral action of the spermicide.

Remember, just because you're not ovulating regularly, don't assume that you're not ovulating at all. To be absolutely safe, all women who could possibly still be fertile should continue using birth control for a full year after their final menstrual period.

3

Symptoms and Solutions

There's an old cartoon that shows a husband returning home from work to find his house in shambles. Garbage is strewn over the floor, laundry is hanging from the lamps and chairs, and the children are chasing each other around the house with guns. His wife looks up from the couch and says, "You know how you're always asking me what I do all day? Well, today I didn't do it."

Estrogen is like the housewife in the cartoon: we don't appreciate all the things it does until it stops doing them. This hormone works behind the scenes to maintain health and vitality, and when it departs from the system, myriad symptoms can occur, ranging from the merely irritating to the severely incapacitating.

When they first begin to appear, perimenopausal symptoms may seem unrelated to each other, and women often treat each problem individually, not seeing the connection until years later. Skipped periods and hot flashes are almost automatically attributed to menopause, but if your first symptom happens to be insomnia or a loss of concentration, you may spend hours in a therapist's office before it becomes apparent that the problem is primarily hormonal. And if your third and fourth symptoms are itchy skin and urinary incontinence, not only are you unlikely to link them to menopause, you're also unlikely to see their connection to the insomnia or concentration loss. A woman may say, "I'm falling apart," failing to recognize that she really has only one condition, perimenopause, that is manifesting itself in many ways.

Perhaps it will help to think of perimenopause as producing a constellation of symptoms. There is a pattern, but you must stand back and take in everything to see it. As long as you focus on each individual star, each individual symptom, you'll miss the bigger picture (see Figure 3.1).

How Bad Will the Symptoms Be?

Most women go through menopause with manageable difficulties, but about 20 percent experience symptoms which they describe as severe enough to affect their functioning at home or work. There's no sure way to predict whether you'll be among the ones who have a rough time, although there is evidence to suggest that thin women have more pronounced symptoms than overweight women. This is due to the fact that fat tissue stores estrogen, allowing for a time-release effect later, and is also capable of manufacturing a weak type of estrogen called estrone, which can curb minor symptoms. Also, as previously discussed, the more abrupt your transition to menopause, the more dramatic your symptoms. In addition, women with a history of PMS or other menstrual difficulties report more problems with menopause than average.

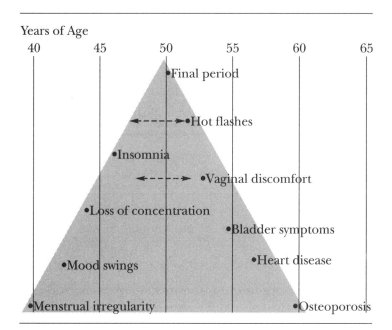

Figure 3.1 Timeline of symptoms in menopause.

HRT: The Umbrella Treatment

A majority of the symptoms we will presently describe respond favorably to hormone replacement therapy, and if your symptoms are bad enough to get you truly down, you should investigate the possibility of HRT even if you're still menstruating. Hormone replacement therapy is a complex and somewhat controversial issue and will be discussed in greater detail in chapters 4 and 5.

For now it is enough to be aware that HRT is the oft-prescribed umbrella treatment for women who are experiencing multiple symptoms, simply because putting estrogen and progesterone back into the system eliminates many complaints in one fell swoop. HRT releases both the doctor and the patient from the arduous task of trying to sort out the causes of individual symptoms. A quick glance at the list of symptoms shows how interrelated many of them are—who can say if she's depressed from a lack of sleep or if she has insomnia because she's depressed? Life's troubles seldom happen in a linear fashion, and since women are subject to such a wide variety of pressures, it can be impossible to say just which symptom came first.

But the interrelationship of the symptoms can also work in your favor, for by solving one problem you often indirectly solve others. Anything that reduces stress reduces the symptoms of perimenopause. Relaxation techniques such as massage, biofeedback, yoga, meditation or prayer, a regular sleep schedule, an exercise program, or even a support group can have a great impact on how you handle perimenopause. Stress-management techniques are proactive medicine in its most potent form: you may not be able to avoid experiencing a single hot flash, but you can stop the domino effect before one symptom, unchecked, sets off another and then another.

Most women who have serious difficulty in perimenopause have multiple symptoms, but a woman experiencing a lone symptom probably won't need the entire battery of HRT to combat it. If insomnia, for example, is the only thing distressing you, try the simple suggestions in the upcoming solution section before embarking on a program designed to relieve a batch of ills you don't have.

Symptoms of Perimenopause

Hot Flashes

The problem: You're sitting at your desk in the midafternoon, when you suddenly feel warm. You remove your jacket and loosen your collar, but within minutes a red flush has risen from your chest and spread across your torso and up your neck to your scalp. You begin sweating, and when you wipe your brow with a tissue, you realize your makeup is coming off. After a couple of uncomfortable minutes and a few pointed glances from the man at the desk beside you, the hot flash abates. But your blouse is soaked with perspiration, and almost immediately you begin to feel chilled.

A whopping 85 percent of menopausal women experience hot flashes. Sometimes called a hot flush, because you redden or blush as a result of the dilation of the blood vessels, a hot flash is a sensation of heat that begins in the face, head, or chest. Some women have a specific focal point such an an earlobe or the skin between their breasts; when they feel the first tingles there, they know a hot flash is approaching. From the initial site, the hot flash can spread over the entire body in a matter of seconds. The degree of sensation varies from mild discomfort to a feeling so intense that women have to fight the urge to pull off clothing.

Hot flashes typically last three minutes but can range in duration from a few seconds to an entire hour. Most menopausal women experience them only for about a year; they are, in fact, one of the more transitory complaints of menopause, and one many women decide simply to bear. But in 25 percent of women they persist for as long as five years—too long to suffer without help.

The precise physical origin of a hot flash is not understood, but it appears to be linked to estrogen withdrawal. Among its many other functions, estrogen affects the hypothalamus, the heat-regulating center in the brain, and as menopause approaches, this internal thermostat gets out of whack. Studies show that a woman's temperature rises slightly just before a hot flash, though you may feel as if it's rising dramatically. One woman described it as the "exploding thermometer effect" of a cartoon. Blood vessels dilate in an attempt to cool the body, causing the flush, and your body begins to sweat in an effort to lower its temperature. Once the flash passes, your pores are open and your skin is damp, setting you up for the chill that frequently follows.

Why are some women affected much more intensely by hot flashes than others? The answer appears to lie in how much their estrogen level varies within the course of a day. If a woman has a small, steady amount of estrogen in her system, her body adapts, but if the levels are continually rising and falling, the body is forced to adjust repeatedly, and hot flashes become more pronounced.

The solution: Estrogen replacement is the foundation of hot flash therapy, dating back to the 19th century when a sheep's ovary sandwich was one prescribed remedy. This is probably where the tradition of "grin and bear it" originated.

Estrogen is now usually administered in either pill or skin-patch form, and its effect on hot flashes is swift. For women who are not good candidates for HRT, the hypertension medicine clonidine has proven to help hot flashes, as have beta-blockers such as Inderal and antiprostaglandins such as naproxen.

If your hot flashes are relatively mild or you'd like to avoid drug therapy, biofeedback has helped some women cope, while a recent European study has shown that women who engage in regular aerobic exercise report only half as many hot flashes as sedentary women. Two things that don't work: Vitamin E was once touted as helpful, but in double-blind studies it was no more effective than a placebo. Barbiturates, often prescribed a generation ago, not only don't stop the flashes from coming but can leave you lethargic and zonked.

Night Sweats and Insomnia

The Problem You awake at 3:15 A.M. in the midst of a hot flash. By the time it passes, your nightgown and sheets are soaked. You get up, shower, change your gown, and put towels over the damp sheets in order not to disturb your husband, but after all this activity, you can't get back to sleep. At 5:21 you're still awake, and since you have to be at work in three hours, you go ahead and get up, knowing you'll drag through the day.

Sweating often follows hot flashes. An episode that occurs at night, called a night sweat, entails an exaggerated feeling of heat, partly because our sleeping bodies beneath their blankets are warmer at night anyway and also because if we're asleep we miss the warning tingles of an approaching flash and are unable to drink water, unbutton our collars or do anything to diminish the impact.

These disturbances can wake you from a sound sleep, and if they happen regularly enough, the result is chronic sleep deprivation, similar to what you experience when a newborn joins the family. Night sweats provide a good example of how one symptom can lead to another; if you go enough nights denied deep sleep, you'll likely become irritable, moody, and prone to locking your keys in your car. Achieving only shallow sleep for a couple of hours at a time is a condition known as low sleep effectiveness. Since older people are at risk for insomnia anyway, a woman plagued with night sweats faces a double whammy: it's harder for her to get to sleep and then harder for her to stay asleep. Untreated, sleep deprivation can lead to depressive disorders.

The solution: HRT helps, because it both reduces the frequency and intensity of hot flashes and improves the general quality of sleep. Regular exercise can effectively battle insomnia, but don't work out within two hours of going to bed or your revved-up metabolism won't allow you to rest. It's also important to practice good sleep hygiene by maintaining a consistent bedtime and engaging in whatever soothing ritual—a warm bath, hot milk, soft music, or reading—works to make you drowsy.

Insomnia is also obviously linked to stress, so any stress-reduction technique, whether yoga, meditation, prayer, or a progressive relaxation tape, will help you get to sleep. Caffeine and alcohol affect people more as they get older, so even if you could have three glasses of wine and then sleep through the night 10 years ago, don't assume that your present wakefulness isn't caused by alcohol. Smoking and some antihistamines have also proven to disrupt the sleep cycle, even in people who did not report sleep problems when they were younger.

If your insomnia does not respond to these common-sense methods, or if HRT stops the night sweats but you're still having trouble getting to sleep, you may need to visit a sleep disorder clinic or try biofeedback. The phone numbers and addresses of the American Sleep Disorders Association and the Biofeedback Society of America are listed in the sources section at the back of this book. These organizations can direct you to the nearest clinic.

Poor Memory and Loss of Concentration

The problem: You notice that you're having trouble remembering simple things, that you have to make a list before going to the supermarket even if you only need three items. Your reaction time seems delayed and you often feel vaguely unfocused.

For a working woman or a mother who has young children depending upon her alertness, memory loss can be among the most upsetting symptoms of perimenopause. Short-term memory is more often affected than long-term. You may look up an address and forget it before you can write it down, or go absolutely blank on the name of your child's third-grade teacher.

One of the reasons memory loss is scary for the menopausal woman is that she may think she's "cracking up" or exhibiting signs of Alzheimer's disease. Even her doctor may not connect her symptoms to estrogen loss, but rather may fuel her fears by attributing the problem to stress or aging. If she's experiencing night sweats and insomnia as well, her troubles with concentration are clearly compounded, as it's hard to stay alert when you've had just four hours of sleep the night before. Once again, the more abrupt the estrogen withdrawal, the more disturbing the symptoms, and women recovering from surgery or chemotherapy often report an alarming degree of forgetfulness, which they generally fail to connect with the loss of their ovaries.

Some slowdown in knowledge retrieval does come with age—for both men and women. You know as much or more as you ever did, but it takes longer to recall the information. A friend of ours who was in the seniors tournament on the TV show "Jeopardy!" explained that older contestants score better than younger ones on the preliminary written test. The seniors haven't forgotten their high school history classes at all and tend to have a wider range of knowledge than the younger contestants. But since older people can't summon the information quite as fast, they're at a disadvantage in the actual game, where speed matters almost as much as knowledge. Hence the show created a separate tournament for people over the age of 50. The questions are just as difficult, but the pace is slightly slower.

For your own peace of mind, it's important to distinguish between perimenopausal forgetfulness and the normal slowdown in information retrieval that comes with age. If you're simply one second slower on the word processor than you used to be, don't worry. This is normal, more than offset by your experience, and shouldn't affect your job performance or self-esteem. But if your short-term memory seems to become drastically worse, or you can't stay with a simple task like a crossword puzzle, your symptoms may be linked to estrogen withdrawal.

The solution: Let's face it: we've all known for years that female hormones make you smarter, and now there's proof. No one understands exactly how estrogen influences brain function, but women who receive HRT report that their concentration and ability to remember things and improve almost immediately.

In addition, anything that helps you achieve deep sleep will lead to improved concentration the next day. Don't hesitate to make lists, to write yourself notes, even to carry a map of your hometown in your car's glove compartment. Most important, relax. You are not getting dumb or going nuts, and this too shall pass.

Menstrual Irregularity

The problem: The night before you leave on a week-long business trip, your period starts. You set out the next day, equipped with tampons and pads, but by the time you arrive, you've stopped bleeding. You wear a pad the next day as a precaution, and by lunch you're bleeding again, this time quite heavily, with cramps. The bleeding lasts only two days, but you keep using the tampons throughout the trip because you're nervous. When you get home, you're aren't sure whether you should even mark the bleeding on your calendar as a period. Who knows when you'll bleed again.

For 1 woman in 10, periods simply stop. But for the other 90 percent, a change in the menstrual cycle is generally a reliable indication of perimenopause.

Unfortunately, there is no way to predict how they will change. Your periods may become shorter, longer, lighter, heavier, closer together, or farther apart. Some women who have never experienced cramps begin to have them, and others who have never experiencd PMS begin to have all the symptoms.

The solution: For starters, chart your bleeding. The first thing that changes is the classic 28-day cycle, and unless you have an accurate record of when and how much you're bleeding, hormone replacement therapy can't help.

Progesterone will regulate your periods, and some HRT regimens stop menstrual bleeding altogether. The pros and cons of the methods will be discussed in the next chapter. Also, if you're still potentially fertile, oral contraceptives will keep your periods regular as well as preventing pregnancy.

Mood Swings

The problem: The dry cleaner tells you he couldn't get the spot out of your blouse, and you burst into tears.

Although this is one of the symptoms most associated with menopause, research has not proven it to be directly connected. The stereotype of the menopausal women sobbing and raging her way through the day finds little support in clinical studies.

Here's what we do know: women are two to three times more likely than men to experience depression, but the onset is most often in the late 30s and early 40s, and more often linked to life changes than hormonal changes. The more severe the depression, the less apt it is to be linked to menopause; while some mood swings can be attributed to fluctuations in your hormone levels, most women report simply feeling on edge or as though they are not coping as well as they used to—not profoundly unhappy.

Also, the women who report depression in menopause often have a history of psychological disorders. If a
woman is teetering on the brink of depression anyway, it's
easy to see how a symptom such as sleep deprivation,
memory loss, or having her period every day of the
month could quickly become the last straw.

Since estrogen and progesterone affect the chemicals
in the brain that regulate appetite as well as sleep and
pain perception, variations in hormone levels can lead to
corresponding fluctuations in how well you're dealing
with the most basic requirements of daily life. It's not that
estrogen deprivation brings you a whole new set of mental
or emotional problems, but it can diminish your capacity
to cope with the problems you already have.

The solution: Anything that improves your general health
will improve your mental outlook. Try following a well-
balanced diet, a regular program of exercise, or vitamin
therapy. HRT can quickly quell the mood swings that
accompany unstable hormone levels, and many women
on HRT report an overall sense of well-being and calm.

If your depression persists, you feel bad all the time
instead of occasionally, or you begin to contemplate suicide, you are not dealing with normal menopausal moodiness. You should see your family physician or a mental
health professional immediately. If your unhappiness is
linked to an unsatisfying job or a troubled relationship, a
therapist or support group can help you make decisions
about your situation. Women in their 40s often feel that
they have to be strong for everyone, especially if they're
caught between the needs of their still-dependent children and imminently dependent parents. Finding someone to listen, be it a counselor or a group of other mid-life
women facing similar changes, can make a huge difference in your outlook.

Some medications can help control anxiety or depression, and these are not the addictive, zombie-making pills

that were routinely doled out to the women of our mothers' generation. Better antidepressants, which don't put you in a stupor or neutralize your ability to make a decision, are available, and you shouldn't hesitate to use them if necessary. Perimenopausal moodiness will pass, but true depression does not, and this is another case in which denying the problem or trying to tough it out will only set you up for a bigger crisis down the road.

Declining Libido

The problem: You wait until you're sure your husband is asleep before you go to bed.

As we've seen, declining levels of estrogen can affect your mood, and consequently your attitude toward sex. In addition, a lack of estrogen leaves the genitals less sensitive to stimulation, so estrogen deprivation alone is enough to damage your libido.

One of the most interesting and little-known facts about the ovary is that it manufactures small amounts of the male hormone, testosterone. Testosterone is the libido hormone for both women and men, and when its production suddenly stops, either through surgical removal of the ovaries or ovarian failure following chemotherapy, your sex drive can drop. (Testosterone production usually continues for several years after estrogen production has ceased, so a hormonally induced loss of libido in natural menopause is rare.)

Before seeking treatment for low sex drive, consider whether your lack of interest might be a secondary symptom of another condition. Are you exhausted from months of interrupted sleep? Are you depressed, especially about aging issues or your relationship with your partner? Have irregular periods or monthlong PMS made you miserable? Most significant, has intercourse become uncomfortable due to vaginal dryness? Anyone will avoid sex if it hurts, and vaginal dryness is a common and treatable problem in perimenopause.

The solution: Sexuality is complex and deeply involved with the mind-body connection. Some women believe, perhaps subconsciously, that age 50 is the automatic end of their sexual selves, and their bodies respond to their minds' grim prediction. The psychology of midlife sexuality will be discussed further in chapter 9.

Declining sexual interest due to falling estrogen levels can be improved with conventional HRT. If, however, your ovaries have been removed or disabled through chemotherapy, HRT can be expanded to include testosterone. This is powerful stuff, so there can be some side effects. But if the dosages are controlled, you should not grow facial hair or develop a lowered voice, despite the horror stories you may have heard. On the plus side, some women report that with just a small amount of testosterone, not only does their sex drive return, but they positively feel like they own the street.

Vaginal Dryness

The problem: You and your husband begin to make love. You think you're aroused, or at least you're mentally excited, but you don't become lubricated. Your husband asks, "Is something wrong?" You say no, because you expect that once intercourse starts you'll loosen up and produce lubrication. Instead, it hurts, almost as if each thrust is tearing your vagina. After just a few seconds your husband doesn't have to ask if anything is wrong. Something clearly is.

As estrogen levels drop, the vaginal lining thins, the walls become dryer and less elastic, and ultimately the vagina itself may even shorten. Intercourse with inadequate lubrication can be uncomfortable enough to induce a woman to avoid sex. If the condition remains untreated to the point where the vagina actually atrophies, intercourse is painful, and in some cases, the vagina has been damaged.

The solution: Vaginal dryness is associated with decreased blood flow to the area, so regular stimulation will keep your vagina more elastic and lubricated. Regular sex and/or masturbation is your first line of defense. If you have a partner, you both need to understand that it may take more foreplay to get you ready for intercourse. Try not to become anxious. If you're tense or negative, discomfort during intercourse can become a self-fulfilling prophecy. Just as your memory retrieval system tends to slow slightly with age, so may your sexual response time, but in both cases the ability is still there. Relax and give yourself time.

If vaginal dryness is your only symptom of perimenopause, you may not require the full HRT package. If you decide to treat this problem as an isolated symptom, you have two options: lubricants or estrogen cream.

Lubricants make sex more comfortable, but don't address the underlying problem, so they are your best bet only if your vaginal dryness is a relatively rare occurance. One popular lubricant is Astroglide, which can be applied right before intercourse; it's light in texture and has no medicinal taste or smell, making it far superior to K-Y Jelly or Vaseline. Another option is Replens, described as a "vaginal moisturizer" rather than a lubricant, which can be applied hours before intercourse. Replens causes the vagina to retain its natural fluid, somewhat like an expensive face cream that causes the skin to plump up temporarily. If used four times a week as directed, Replens frequently restores moisture to the degree that an additional lubricant is not needed, and many women prefer it for this reason. Of course, Astro-glide does have a far more exciting name.

If your vaginal dryness is chronic or pronounced, your doctor will more likely prescribe an estrogen cream. In comparison to oral estrogen or skin patches, these vaginal creams supply little estrogen—sufficient to lubricate the vagina but not to protect against heart disease and osteo-porosis or to quell hot flashes. But just as the creams pro-vide fewer of the benefits of estrogen, they also carry fewer of the risks, and they have the advantage of working rapidly to restore vaginal moisture.

In even more severe cases—if the vagina has begun to shrink or tear, for example—full-scale HRT will be neces-sary to restore vaginal function. Unfortunately, it may take several months on oral or transdermal estrogen for the vagina to regain its elasticity and moisture. In the mean-time, a vaginal hormone cream can prompt lubrication and make intercourse more appealing. Within a few months your vagina will have begun to respond to the HRT and you'll be able to stop using the cream.

Vaginal dryness has two more bothersome side effects. First, even if sex doesn't hurt, a woman in estrogen with-drawal may find that her tissues are less sensitive to stimu-lation. The second unwelcome complication is an increase in minor vaginal infections. HRT helps both con-ditions. If you are prone to vaginal infections, wearing cot-ton panties, sleeping with no underwear, and avoiding the prolonged use of tampons should help you prevent them.

Urinary Incontinence

The problem: You sneeze and you wet yourself.

There are two kinds of urinary problems associated with perimenopause. Some women simply lose control, and a small amount of urine is released whenever they laugh, cough, or sneeze. The reason is that the muscles around the bladder and urethra are lax. Ordinarily, the vaginal wall provides support for the bladder, but as it weakens, either due to repeated childbearing or estrogen deprivation, the bladder can drop out of place. Without the support of the vaginal wall and the muscles surrounding the bladder, even the slight pressure of a single cough can trigger a loss of urine.

The second problem is frequent, painful, or urgent urination. A woman may feel as if she has to urinate all the time, even though her mad dash to the rest room results in only a few drops. The urethra has receptors for estrogen, and without this hormone, the urethra can atrophy much like the vagina. The walls become thinner, weaker, and more likely to develop infections.

The solution: If your condition is due to slack muscles, you may be able to turn the condition around with Kegels. These are rhythmic exercises, named after the doctor who developed them, that are usually suggested to new mothers for restoring muscle tone following childbirth. A Kegel is simply a tightening and releasing motion, as if you were trying to stop the flow of urine. (In fact, if you have trouble getting the hang of them, you may want to practice by stopping the release of urine while on the toilet, letting it start again, stopping it again, etc., until you're familiar with what the muscle contraction feels like.)

The Kegel is a small, subtle movement, and the key to success is to do many of them. Begin with 10 and work up to 10 sets of 10. Women who are most successful with Kegels find a way to incorporate them into their daily routine; they do them when they're on the phone, in the car, or watching the nightly news.

This condition can be persistent, and some women need more help. Since urinary tract infections are a frequent side effect of stress incontinence, you should be evaluated and treated for any infections first. Estrogen, especially if administered in the form of vaginal cream, is a direct approach to the problem. HRT will thicken and tone both the vaginal wall and the urethra, while improving the results from your Kegels regimen.

If your pelvic relaxation is too advanced to respond to HRT, surgical correction may be necessary. But beware of the doctor who advises an operation without giving HRT and Kegels a try; demand a cystometrogram to evaluate your bladder function before agreeing to surgery.

Headaches

The problem: Your head hurts. It feels like a premenstrual migraine—except you're having them once a week.

Sometimes rising and falling estrogen levels cause headaches. Women who were prone to premenstrual migraines are especially likely to experience perimenopausal headaches. HRT can also be a culprit; when women begin HRT, their hormone levels jump rather erratically, resulting in headaches which, while temporary, can be intense.

The solution: If you're prone to headaches and on HRT, consider using the skin patch instead of pills. The patch allows a more steady absorption of the hormone, which may prevent the headaches.

Anything that triggered a migraine in your premenopausal days—certain foods, alcohol, poor sleep, stress—is apt to trigger one now. Regular exercise reduces the incidence of headaches, and biofeedback has been a boon for many migraine sufferers. If all else fails, your physician can prescribe pain medication.

Joint Aches and Back Pains

The problem: You have a constant dull backache, somewhat like the ones you used to get before your periods would start.

Joint and back pain is an occasional secondary complaint of perimenopause, even among women who do not have a history of joint disease or arthritis.

The solution: Regular exercise helps, especially yoga and stretching, which can maintain and improve joint flexibility. Learn your moves in a class with a qualified instructor, however. Improperly done, stretches can cause more injuries than they prevent. HRT also eases joint aches, although no one is sure why.

Joint aches can be a fairly inconspicuous complaint. Some women don't realize they were having them until they begin HRT for another reason and suddenly find it easier to garden or play tennis.

Dry Skin, Wrinkling, and Itching

The problem: Your skin has begun to sag and wrinkle. You feel that you look significantly older than you did last year.

Skin wrinkling occurs as we age for many reasons, most notably sustained exposure to the sun and the gradual loss of collagen, the protein responsible for skin's elasticity and tone. Only recently have we begun to fully understand the role estrogen plays in collagen production, but studies have shown that menopausal women on estrogen have thicker skin with a higher collagen content than women who do not take estrogen.

A very small percentage of women experience a problem that make wrinkles seem like a party. Formication is a sensation like bugs are crawling on your skin, a persistent itchiness or tingling that goes far beyond the normal irritation of dry skin. Fortunately, this is a rare symptom, and one that responds well to HRT.

The solution: Women's magazines have published numerous articles on good skin care, illustrating the dangers of sun exposure and debating the merits of the plentiful collagen-replacement products on the market. Some women opt for cosmetic surgery. However, many plastic surgeons will not perform a face-lift on a woman who is not on HRT, so vital is estrogen to the healing and health of skin. Surgery can lift the skin back into position, but without the elasticity that comes with adequate estrogen, the long-term benefits of a face-lift are reduced and the skin begins to sag again much more quickly. While no one is suggesting that you undergo HRT strictly for cosmetic reasons, more youthful skin is an undeniable side benefit of hormone replacement.

4

❧

Hormone Replacement Therapy

The use of hormone replacement therapy is one of the most controversial aspects of menopause, as reflected in the fact that while 85 percent of doctors advocate HRT, only 20 percent of American women over the age of 50 are currently following their advice. Why do so few women opt for HRT? Possibly because they have so many unanswered questions: Should you engage in a therapy that reduces your chance of a heart attack but may increase your risk for breast cancer? How do you wade through all the potential dosing regimens to find the right one? Will you still have periods? Is HRT something you do for a couple of years until the hot flashes abate, or is this a decision for life?

In this chapter, we'll look at the benefits and drawbacks of hormone replacement therapy, discuss the most common types of medication used, and address the concerns women have. The goal is neither to preach nor frighten, but to give you enough information so you can participate in an informed discussion with your physician about what's right for you.

Natural Versus Medicated Menopause

For some women, the debate on HRT is over before it begins, since they have a philosophical aversion to medical intervention in a natural process. Here we respond to some of the most common protests against HRT.

Argument
It's not natural.

Rebuttal
Frankly, it's not natural to live this long. A century ago, diseases such as polio and diphtheria wiped out a certain percentage of the population before it reached adulthood. Childbirth was much more hazardous. Those women who made it to menopause were considered elderly, not expected to live more than a decade past "the change." But since our generation will on average survive into our 80s, what will happen to the American health-care system if this huge block of women becomes incapacitated by heart disease and osteoporosis? Does it make sense to use medicine to extend the length of life but not to improve the quality of life?

Remember what the *R* in HRT stands for. This therapy is not adding something new. It's *replacing* what the body was once able to produce naturally for itself with a synthetic version. A woman taking estrogen is like a diabetic taking insulin: she's putting back what was was lost, not introducing something utterly foreign into her system.

Argument
My mother didn't do it.

Rebuttal
That's a rather flimsy argument. If you are a woman of the baby boomer generation, by this point in your life you have likely done many things that your mother didn't do.

If your family follows the statistical norm, your mother will not live as long as you will live. Our grandmothers may have considered themselves elderly at 50 and our mothers may have considered themselves old at that age; but now 50 is described as mid-life. A different life expectancy calls for a different health-care strategy.

While we're on the issue of expectancy, it's also possible that you mother simply didn't expect to feel as good as you expect to feel. The women currently approaching menopause have very high expectations of their energy level and ability to cope with daily life. Your mother may indeed have survived menopause without any intervention, but if her symptoms were severe she simply endured them, figuring that this was just the way women typically felt after the age of 50.

Argument
I'm afraid of the side effects, especially the increased risk of cancer.

Rebuttal:
HRT does indeed entail risks, though there are also risks that come with not taking HRT. The pluses and minuses will be analyzed more fully in the next chapter, but the point is that each woman sitting around the table has been dealt a different genetic hand, and she will have to adjust her strategy to fit the particular cards she holds. Look at your family and individual medical history. A woman with a predisposition toward osteoporosis may make a different decision than a woman with a history of breast cancer.

Argument
I don't understand it.

Rebuttal
HRT is complicated but comprehensible. You're already making a start by reading up on the subject, and the next step is to find a doctor who will take the time to explain your options and address your concerns.

What is lacking, not only for HRT but for all the issues of menopause, is a readily accessible pool of information, like the one we currently have in place for childbirth. When a woman, for example, decides she wants to try to deliver her second child vaginally after having the first via cesarean section, there's a name for this. She's seeking a "VBAC," a vaginal birth after cesarean. With a few phone calls, she should able to find a support group, a handful of books on the subject, and a list of physicians and mid-wives in her area with experience in this type of delivery. A woman suffering severe vaginal dryness and atrophy in menopause is certainly in need of the same support, but it's highly unlikely she'll find any system in place to help her, much less a ready-made group of sympathetic friends and sensitized doctors to see her through the condition.

We need to establish far more information and support systems for women who are having a tough time with menopause. In the meantime, keep reading, find a good doctor, and look for lectures or support groups sponsored by area hospitals. HRT is ultimately a decision you'll make by yourself, but don't make it in the absence of information.

Argument
My symptoms aren't that bad.

Rebuttal
For many women, symptoms aren't severe and can be handled with the passage of time or the natural remedies

outlined in chapter 7. But women without harsh symptoms should still consider the issue of long-term health risks. If you have a family history of heart disease or osteoporosis, HRT is worth investigating, even if you never feel a single hot flash.

Argument:
It's just not me.

Rebuttal
You'll get no argument from us on this one.

Women need to bind together for some purposes: to bring attention to the health-care issues our generation faces as we age, to make information more readily available, to support that percentage of us who will suffer pronounced menopausal distress, and to insist that more dollars are spent on research into "women's diseases" such as breast cancer and osteoporosis.

But the bottom line is that, like other sexual/reproductive issues, HRT is intensely personal. As with the issue of abortion, how you feel about it politically and what you might do personally could well be two different things. As mid-life women lobby to be taken seriously by the medical community, we stand as a group, but when it comes time to either take that pill or not take it, each woman stands alone. Try not to base your decision on a philosophical agenda. Instead, base it on your personal risk factors, the severity of your symptoms, and your tolerance for physicians, medications, and routines in general.

What Does HRT Do?

HRT effectively treats hot flashes, vaginal dryness, and urinary incontinence. Insomnia and moodiness improve, as does memory and concentration. Periods become regular and lighter. Many women, freed from these problems, report that their energy returns to previous levels. Estrogen dramatically increases your protection against heart disease and bone loss. There are cosmetic benefits as well. Many women consider estrogen to be a type of youth drug, producing more elastic skin and shinier hair.

Obviously, any woman's life could be improved by the list above, but the need is greater for some women than for others. You should seriously consider hormone therapy if:

♦ Menopause is making you miserable. Your symptoms are affecting your quality of life.

♦ You've had an oophorectomy, undergone chemotherapy, or for some reason have been thrown into an earlier menopause than is typical.

♦ You have heart disease or are at high risk for it.

♦ You have osteoporosis or are at high risk for it.

Why Don't Women Stay with It?

At the beginning of this chapter we noted that the percentage of physicians who recommend HRT is much larger than the percentage of women who use HRT. Perhaps an even more unsettling statistic is that 20 percent of the women why try HRT stop within nine months—and that's probably a lowball figure because many women who don't like HRT simply never return to their physicians and their experiences are thus not entered into the statistics. Most of the women who throw in the towel do so because of side effects such as bloating, break-through bleeding, or nausea. A lucky few achieve the perfect combination immediately, but for most women, HRT involves as much as a year of fiddling, and several visits to the physician.

Most likely, after trying your first regimen for three months, you'll revisit the doctor to discuss side effects and complications. At this point, changes may be made in the dosage, the brand of medication, or the method of administration. After you've found a combination that produces either few or no unpleasant side effects, the next visit, which usually is scheduled six to nine months after HRT is started, is to see whether you are still doing well; you may need further alterations in dosage. The aim of responsible HRT is to find the most effective dose for each woman, low enough to minimize side effects while still high enough to treat her symptoms and protect her from heart disease and osteoporosis. Eventually, within 18 months, you should have found what works for you and your subsequent visits to your doctor can just be for annual exams.

So even in an ideal scenario, a woman should plan on three to five office visits to regulate her HRT. Some women have to be far more persistent. We interviewed one woman who tried 15 different drugs before she got relief. Obviously, if you're going to be seeing your physician this frequently and putting a good deal of faith in his or her judgment, it's essential to have the right doctor. In chapter 8, we discuss how to find someone who will listen and take the time to fine-tune your particular therapy. Without a doctor who understands the process of HRT, your chances of successful therapy diminish and you're much more likely to become one of the women who give up on it too soon.

How Much Is Enough?

HRT has three goals:

♦ to treat acute symptoms such as hot flashes and night sweats

♦ to treat intermediate symptoms such as vaginal dryness and urinary incontinence

♦ to provide long-term health protection against coronary disease and bone loss

Estradiol is the predominant form of estrogen produced by the ovary before menopause, and estradiol levels vary from 40 pg/ml (picogram/milliliter) to 400
pg/ml during a typical menstrual cycle. After menopause,
levels fall to approximately 20 pg/ml. Generally, a blood
level of 50 to 65 pg/ml will cure symptoms and protect
the heart and bones. Some women will require higher levels to feel their best, but the goal is to use the lowest dose
that gets the job done.

Women who had problems with birth control pills
sometimes assume that they're not good candidates for
HRT, but the dosage of estrogen required to suppress ovulation is three to five times higher than that required to
relieve the symptoms of menopause. Thus, many women
who avoided the Pill because of problems such as blood
clots can probably take HRT. If you have memories of
weight gain and bloating while on the Pill, don't automatically rule out HRT: lower dosages also mean fewer side
effects.

What Are the Risks of HRT?

Side effects of taking estrogen include nausea, headaches,
and bloating. The dosage and the method of taking the
medicine may influence the degree to which you experience the effects. Progesterone, the hormone that brings
on your periods, is often a component of HRT and can
produce PMS-like symptoms such as fluid retention,
moodiness, breast tenderness, and headaches.

Beyond side effects, there are long-term health risks
for some women. HRT can cause hypertension, liver and
blood-clotting problems, and, as will be discussed in the
next chapter, may increase your risk of breast cancer. You
are a poor candidate for HRT if:

♦ You have been previously diagnosed with breast cancer.

♦ You have blood clots or phlebitis.

♦ You have had endometrial cancer.

♦ You have uterine fibroids.

♦ You have had gallbladder or liver disease.

The last two items on the list require a judgment call; many women with gallbladder or liver disease can still take HRT, but they should be monitored especially closely. Women with liver disease will probably want to opt for the patch method, which allows estrogen to be absorbed directly into the bloodstream without being processed by the liver, instead of taking estrogen in pill form.

The majority of uterine fibroids, those benign tumors that affect more than 25 percent of women over 35, do not require treatment; in fact, many women who have fibroids are unaware of it. Sometimes, however, fibroids can cause abdominal discomfort or heavy menstrual bleeding. The standard treatment used to be hysterectomy, but new procedures allow doctors to remove the fibroids or shrink them with drugs, while leaving the uterus intact. For most women, the amount of estrogen in HRT is not enough to affect their fibroids, but some tumors are more sensitive to estrogen than others. The typical treatment is to begin HRT if needed, monitor the fibroids on a regular basis, and discontinue the HRT if they appear to be growing.

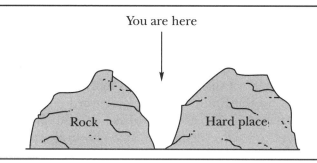

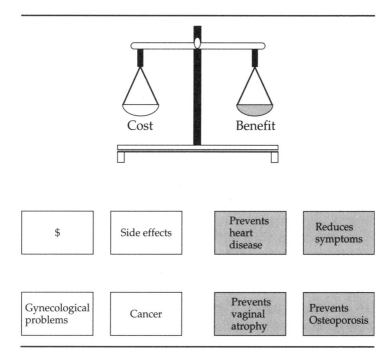

Figure 4.1 Estrogen Replacement Therapy Costs and Benefits

How Many Hormones Will I Have to Take?

If you've had a hysterectomy, and thus have no risk of uterine cancer, you can take estrogen alone. Estrogen increases your risk of endometrial cancer, so women who still have a uterus should add progestin, the synthetic form of the hormone progesterone, to their regimen; the inclusion of progesterone to estrogen eliminates the added risk of endometrial cancer. (It's a bit confusing, but progesterone, the natural hormone, is difficult to absorb, so what is usually prescribed in HRT is the synthetic form. In the future, we'll use the word *progesterone* when referring to the natural substance and *progestin* when referring to the drug that acts like progesterone when administered to the body.)

Provera is the brand name of the most commonly pre-scribed progestin and Premarin is the most commonly prescribed estrogen. This classic combination has even earned a nickname, the P and P Cocktail. Many physicians will first try 0.625 mg of Premarin and 10 mg of Provera daily for 10 to 12 days a month, but if this standard dose doesn't work to relieve your symptoms or causes uncomfortable side effects, don't despair. There are certainly other combinations.

Will I Still Have Periods?

With estrogen alone, there is no period. Progesterone, however, is the hormone that rises after ovulation in a fertile woman to build up the endometrium and, if she has not conceived, ultimately falls and brings on her period. When combined with estrogen in a menopausal woman, it encourages her body to mimic the monthly cycle.

Depending on how you feel about having a period, there are two basic ways to take the medication: cyclically, which causes periods, or continuously, which keeps you from having periods.

The cyclic method involves taking estrogen on days 1 through 25, and progestin on days 14 through 25. On the 26th day of the month, you stop taking both hormones and then have a period. For most women, the bleeding eventually becomes predictable and light, somewhat like the periods you have when you've been on the Pill for a year or two.

In continuous therapy, you take lower dosages of progestin—say, 2.5 mg of Provera daily instead of the standard 5 or 10 mg—but you take both the estrogen and progestin every day of the month. There are no days when you're off medication, ergo, no bleeding.

So why doesn't every woman opt to be period-free? The problem with continuous therapy is break-through bleeding, and many women prefer the predictable period of the cyclic method to the random bleeding of continuous therapy. If you're willing to persist with the continuous method, however, most women manage to eliminate all bleeding within a year.

Dosing Regimens

It's not just what you take, it's also when you take it and what else you're taking with it. HRT encompasses several dosing regimens. Some of the most common are analyzed below.

Cyclic Estrogen

Although rarely used today, cyclic estrogen was popular in the mid-1970s. A woman would take 21 to 25 days of "unopposed," or straight, estrogen, causing little, if any, uterine bleeding, even during the 5 to 9 days in which she wasn't taking the hormone.

Scientists have since learned that unopposed estrogen increases the risk of endometrial cancer, but even for a woman without a uterus, cyclic estrogen may not be the best method. She may redevelop her menopausal symptoms during the days off estrogen and require the first week of the next month's therapy just to regain her footing. There's no real advantage to cyclic estrogen, which pretty much represents the dinosaur days of HRT.

Continuous Estrogen

If a woman doesn't have a uterus, she can take unopposed estrogen every day of the month, usually in the form of pills or skin patches.

Note: It has been proven that progestin reduces the risk of uterine cancer, but some experts argue that it also cuts the risk of breast cancer, making it beneficial even to the woman who has had a hysterectomy. There's no conclusive evidence of this yet, but if it is proven, progestin may become part of every woman's HRT regimen.

Cyclic Estrogen plus Cyclic Progestin

Estrogen is given daily for the first 25 days of the month with progestin added for the last 12 days of this time. (Administration is often adjusted to fit individual needs; progestin may be required for as few as 10 or as many as 14 days to regulate bleeding.) After the 25th day, both hormones are stopped, and the woman will have a light period. As with cyclic estrogen, the disadvantage to this program is that symptoms may recur during the 5 to 6 days without estrogen.

Continuous Estrogen plus Cyclic Progestin

This is the regimen recommended by most menopause experts. A good choice for women with acute symptoms, it involves a daily administration of estrogen, with progestin added for 12 days of the month. Since you never go off the estrogen, your symptoms never recur, but using the progestin in cyclic dosage means you'll still have a period. Which 12 days you take the progestin—and hence, when you have your period—is up to you; your period begins as soon as the progestin part of the therapy winds down. If you don't want to always have your period during end-of-the-month holidays like Thanksgiving and Christmas, start taking your progestin on the first day of the month, and your period will begin around the 13 to 15th day of the month.

For women who take estrogen via the skin patch, the system is similar. A patch lasts basically three days, so after you've gone through four patches, add the progestin in pill form. Keep changing the patches twice a week throughout the month, since the estrogen is continuous, but discontinue the progestin after 12 days, and you'll have your period.

Continuous Estrogen plus Continuous Progestin

This regimen was developed for women who wish to avoid the withdrawal bleeding or periods that begin when you stop taking progestin. Both estrogen and progestin are taken daily, the Provera in a lower dose (2.5 mg).

As previously mentioned, women starting out with this regimen commonly experience irregular break-through bleeding for six to nine months. But if you can stick it out until the progestin dosage is fine-tuned, this program usually stops periods altogether within a year. Continuous estrogen and progestin seems to work best for women who have been postmenopausal for more than one year —who are more rarely bothered with break-through bleeding. One note: This method hasn't been around as long as the continuous estrogen and cyclic progestin regimen, so the long-term effects have not been studied as thoroughly.

Continuous Progestin Alone

For women who can't take estrogen, continous progestin has been shown to relieve hot flashes and may prevent bone loss. It has no heart benefits, however, and doesn't help vaginal or urogenital symptoms.

Types of Estrogen

Premarin

This commonly used form is purified from the urine of pregnant mares, hence the name. Typical doses are 0.625 mg and 1.25 mg. Higher doses of 2.5 mg and 5.0 mg are available but rarely used.

17b-Estradiol

This is the predominant form of estrogen produced by the ovaries before menopause. It is available in both oral (brand name: Estrace) and transdermal (brand name: Estraderm) forms. The transdermal form bypasses the liver, and in the oral form the liver converts 17b-Estradiol to estrone (a weaker estrogen) before it is released into general circulation. The usual dose is 1 to 2 mg, but the FDA has approved a smaller dosage of 0.5 mg for prevention of bone loss. A dosage of less than 1 mg usually doesn't relieve symptoms but is a good option for a postmenopausal woman whose symptoms have long since abated and who is looking to estrogen only for its long-term health benefits.

Estrone Conjugate

This is a derivative of the predominant form of estrogen produced by the postmenopausal ovary, effective both for relieving symptoms and preventing bone loss. Brand names are Ogen and Ortho EST. Some women find they have less menstrual flow on HRT with Estrone Conjugate than with other forms of estrogen.

If you can't take estrogen, clonidine (brand name: Catapres) is a good substitute for relieving symptoms, although it does not offer the long-term health benefits of estrogen.

Methods of Administration

Currently in the United States, estrogen can be given via pill, patch, cream, or injection. Each method has its pros and cons.

Oral

After being broken down by the intestinal tract and processed by the liver, all oral forms of estrogen essentially produce the same end product, estrone, which circulates in the blood and relieves symptoms. Common brand names of oral estrogen are Premarin, Estrace, Ogen, and Ortho EST.

Pluses: Many women are used to taking medication in pill form, and it's not hard to make a pill part of your daily routine. The pills are neat and easy to pack when traveling; most important, it's simple to alter dosage level if need be.

Minuses: Estrogens increase the liver's production of clotting factors, which theoretically could place a woman at risk for deep vein thrombosis. This same risk accompanied the Pill in the 1970s—the possibility of blood clots was a drawback for some women. It's worth remembering, however, that HRT uses a much smaller dosage of estrogen than the Pill and has a correspondingly lower risk for clotting disorders. Unless you have a personal history of thrombosis or blood clots, this is probably not a problem for you.

In addition, some women develop hypertension on oral estrogens in response to the increased renin activity in the liver.

Less serious side effects include nausea and bloating. Using Estrace under the tongue may reduce these symptoms while still enabling you to use a pill. Also, taking estrogen at bedtime seems to lessen the sensation of nausea, or at least delay it until you're asleep and unaware.

Transdermal

Patches containing 17b-estradiol in a reservoir are applied to the skin where they provide relatively constant serum levels for approximately 84 hours. You change the patch every three to four days. This method allows the estrogen to be absorbed into the bloodstream without being initially processed by the liver.

The patch comes in two sizes or doses, 0.05 mg and 0.1 mg, representing the amount of estradiol delivered to the patient through the skin each day. In Europe, a 0.025 mg patch is used for starting women on estrogen more slowly and gently and reducing side effects such as breast tenderness. This dosage is currently unavailable in the U.S., but by placing a round Band-Aid under the 0.05 patch, you can reduce the amount of estradiol that passes through to the skin and create the same low-dosage effect.

Pluses: Many women like the patch because they don't have to think about it. The gradual, constant absorption of estrogen mutes symptoms and creates few side effects, and the fact that the patch method bypasses the liver is a plus for women with a history of liver disease. And, like pills, it is easy to change the dosage level if needed.

Minuses: The patch adheres to the skin via a layer of adhesive; some women are allergic to this or develop skin irritation. Spraying Vancenase (a corticosteroid developed for intranasal use) on the skin prior to applying the patch has been reported to reduce skin irritation. The patch adheres well enough during showering or swimming, but may not stay on for prolonged soaks. If you're planning to get into a hot tub or swim the English Channel, you can always remove the patch and replace it after your skin is dry.

Sweating can also unstick the patch. Women who live in hot, humid climate, and athletes who perspire heavily often report that the patches become loosened. Applying paper tape, which is available in drugstores, can help hold the patch in place.

Some women simply do not absorb the estradiol from the patch. If a woman continues to have menopausal symptoms while on the patch, especially on the bigger 0.1 patch, her serum estradiol level should be checked.

The last complaint is rather trivial. Occasionally a woman's sexual partner will complain about the aesthetics of the patch, which is generally placed on the hip or thigh. If this is a problem, you may want to change your method of administration—or your partner.

Vaginal Cream

Estrogen in cream form can be inserted directly into the vagina, which is especially useful in treating vaginal dryness. Don't wait until the situation worsens before seeking help. It takes a long time to overcome a dry or atrophied vagina; even if you're taking HRT via the oral or patch form, it may be necessary to supplement this with the cream in order to relubricate your vagina.

Vaginal creams are available in Premarin, Ogen, and Estrace preparations. Some estrogen is absorbed through the vaginal epithelium (lining) into the systemic circulation, but this amount isn't enough to prevent heart disease and bone loss. Usually one-quarter of an applicator daily for four weeks is adequate, with booster doses a couple of times a week after that. Within a few months, the pill or patch estrogen alone will be enough to alleviate the dry vagina and use of the cream can be dropped.

Pluses: Creams are by far the quickest way to treat vaginal dryness—the perfect local treatment for a local problem.

Minuses: The creams can be messy, and it's hard to control the dosage with precision. While the creams don't contain enough estrogen to offer long-term health benefits, sometimes enough is absorbed into the bloodstream to affect other organs, such as the breast or uterus. Thus a woman who can't take estrogen in oral or patch form may find herself developing the same adverse side effects with the creams, albeit to a lesser degree. Also, the creams should not be used just prior to intercourse. A man can absorb enough estrogen through his penis to cause side effects such as breast enlargement.

Note: A somewhat unusual but workable alternative for patients who don't tolerate oral estrogen or who have skin irritations from the patch is to insert Estrace tablets into the vagina. Adequate medication is absorbed to provide the heart and bone benefits, and the dosage is controlled more easily than with cream preparations.

Injections

Estradiol preparations can be administered intramuscularly, usually once a month.

Pluses: You don't have to think about it.

Minuses: You can't remove the medication once it has been injected, even if side effects develop. Also, a woman's tolerance may rise, forcing the physician to use increasingly higher dosages to achieve the same effects.

On the Horizon

These methods of application are not currently available for general use in the U.S., but are offered in Europe and may have won FDA approval by the time you need them.

Pellet   Crystalline 17b-estradiol pellets can be implanted under the skin, so the estrogen is absorbed directly into the bloodstream, bypassing the liver. The pellets can remain in place for up to six months until the patient needs another insertion. Insertion of the pellets is a minor surgical procedure, done under local anesthesia.

Pluses: For six months, you really don't have to think about HRT. Also, since the liver doesn't process the estrogen, this is a good option for women with liver problems.

Minuses: The pellets can be difficult to remove if the woman is experiencing troublesome side effects. In addition, some women develop a tolerance for the high levels of estradiol in the pellets, necessitating more frequent placement of the pellets and/or higher doses.

Vaginal Rings   The ring, once inserted into the top of the vagina, will gradually release estrogen for up to three months.

Pluses: The ring can easily be removed if a problem develops, or for routine cleaning. Because of the time-release effect, serum levels of estrogen remain consistent as long as the ring is in place.

Minuses: The rings are not currently approved for use in the U.S.

Skin Creams and Gels   17b-estradiol gel, currently popular in France, can be applied to the abdomen and absorbed through the skin.

Pluses: The gels are a no-fuss, noninvasive way to relieve minor symptoms.

Minuses: They are messy to apply, and achieving precise dosages is difficult.

Types of Progestin

While progestin doesn't come in as many forms as estrogen, you still have options.

Most women choose the pill form, but "pure" progestin is poorly absorbed when taken orally. High dosages, such as 200 mg two times a day, are required; since progesterone makes many women drowsy, 300 mg taken before bedtime is a common alternative to the twice-a-day regimen. The pills can also be placed directly into the vagina.

One brand of progestin, Provera, is so commonly prescribed that *Provera* and *progestin* are often used interchangeably. Other brand names include Cycrin, Curretab, and Amen, while generic Provera is called medroxyprogesterone acetate, or MPA.

Daily Provera dosages range from 2.5 mg to 10 mg, and the side effects of this bring-on-the-blood hormone, not surprisingly, are similar to premenstrual symptoms—bloating, sore breasts, irritability, and slight weight gain. You may think your PMS has been reincarnated. The symptoms increase over the course of administration; if you take the hormone for 12 days, you'll have more pronounced symptoms on day 10 than on day one.

Progesterone can also be taken in the form of vaginal or rectal suppositories. The suppositories must be used twice daily and are predictably messy. Injections of progesterone don't work well for HRT; the shots are painful and have to be administered often.

In Great Britain, promising testing is being done on a progestin patch, using a progestin derivative of testosterone called norethindrone. Norethindrone, which is sold under the brand names NOR-QD and Micronor, is already used in the U.S. in oral contraceptives; it protects the endometrium from cancer just as well as Provera. Just as with estrogen, the progestin patch seems to provide a more gradual absorption of the hormone, producing fewer PMS-like side effects than the pills.

Testosterone Replacement

In addition to estrogen and progesterone, the premenopausal ovary produces androgens, a group of "male" hormones that includes testosterone. In fact, the ovary continues to generate small amounts of testosterone even after production of estrogen and progesterone has shut down, but since these levels are not as high as they were before menopause, it makes sense that some women might benefit from androgen replacement.

Testosterone not only boosts the libido but also decreases the anxiety and depression some women suffer in perimenopause. Women who undergo removal of their ovaries prior to menopause particularly benefit from testosterone replacement, since the sudden withdrawal of hormones often leads to an equally sudden drop in their sex drive. If these women are given estrogen, their hot flashes and night sweats may disappear, but they often complain that "something" is still missing. Testosterone replacement turns the lights back on—increasing energy, libido, and general optimism.

Furthermore, testosterone reduces breast tenderness for both women who recently began HRT and perimenopausal women who suffer this symptom before menstruation. As an added bonus, testosterone also helps prevent bone loss.

But many women worry about the side effects. Although some experience mild acne and a degree of hair growth, testosterone dosage levels are quite low and very few women report overtly masculine changes such as a deeper voice. Some physicians have speculated that administering testosterone to women would cause their LDL levels to rise and their HDL levels to fall, putting them at increased risk of heart disease. But studies on women who take testosterone haven't shown the hormone to have an adverse effect on their blood-plasma cholesterol levels.

Testosterone can be administered either by injection or by pill. The injection (brand: Depo-Testadiol) is a combination of estradiol and testosterone given every four to six weeks. The pill, (brand name: Estratest) combines estrogen and testosterone and can be taken every day or alternated with estrogen every other day, depending upon whether the woman develops side effects.

Testosterone replacement isn't necessary for everyone, but for women who have lost their ovaries abruptly due to surgery or any woman troubled by declining sexual energy, it can be an important component of HRT.

Is HRT Forever?

How long a woman should take HRT depends upon her goals for therapy. If relief of hot flashes and night sweats is her primary concern, she may only need to take HRT for a couple of years and then be gradually weaned off the medication. Vaginal dryness and atrophy usually require longer treatment, but in general a woman using HRT to reduce menopausal symptoms should need HRT for only two to four years.

If you're looking for heart or bone benefits, the perspective changes. The moment a woman goes off HRT, bone loss will resume at the same accelerated rate typical of menopause. Less is known about the prevention of heart disease, but women who have been on estrogen for 10 years or longer have markedly less heart disease than women who took estrogen for a short time. If you are at high risk for either heart or bone disease, you should consider staying on estrogen for life.

Both you and your physician should be flexible in your approach, not only when deciding whether to use HRT but also when determining how long to continue it.

5

~~~~

Risky Business: Heart Disease, Osteoporosis, and Breast Cancer

You may not believe it when you're in the middle of a hot flash, but the symptoms of perimenopause can be your best friends. We all nod sagely when the local newscast runs a special on making lifestyle changes to prevent illness, but, human nature being what it is, we are far less motivated by the threat of the serious health problem 20 years away than we are by the immediate discomfort of the symptom at hand.

Hot flashes and irregular bleeding are the irritants that drive women into their doctors' offices and force them to confront the long-term effects of menopause. Perimenopause can serve as the wake-up call that impels a woman to make the changes she's been talking about making for decades, and while we may not be delighted when the alarm goes off, we're actually lucky to have a built-in hormonal impetus to get us moving. The wake-up call for men is usually a heart attack.

The three major diseases facing women as they age are heart disease, osteoporosis, and cancer. Hormone replacement therapy, the standard cure for most menopausal symptoms, reduces a woman's risk for heart disease and bone loss but may increase her risk for cancer, especially breast cancer. In a perfect world, all would be clear and the same prescription would suffice for everyone, but it seems that once hormones enter the picture, nothing is ever perfectly clear again. "What finally makes up your mind about estrogen," said one woman we interviewed, "comes down to what disease you most fear." Let's look at the three big health fears women face as they age and examine how the conventional means of treatment affects an individual's risk for each.

Heart Disease

The problem: Heart disease is the number one killer of women over 50, who, in fact, have twice as high a chance of dying of heart disease as of any kind of cancer. But because the medical community considers heart attacks to be a "male problem," coronary disease in women is underfinanced, underresearched, and underdiagnosed.

Estrogen and progesterone protects women from the hardening of the arteries that precedes many kinds of heart disease, and during the years in which these hormones are in our system, we have a far lower chance of developing heart attacks than men do. But when we lose these vital hormones, our risk of cardiovascular disease rises sharply, particularly the risk of strokes.

Partly because women develop heart disease later than men, we are less likely to be diagnosed and treated. The majority of the large, federally funded studies on heart disease have been conducted in Veterans Administration hos-

Risk Factors for Heart Disease

1. Do you suffer from hypertension?
2. Do you have a family history of heart disease?
3. Are you obese? *(Obesity* is defined as weighing 20 percent more than the charts recommend. If your ideal weight is 120 and you weigh 145, you're crossing the line from a cosmetic problem to a health one.)
4. Do you have a sedentary lifestyle?
5. Do you smoke?
6. Are you under a lot of stress?
7. Are you diabetic?
8. Do you have unfavorable plasma lipid levels, i.e., high total cholesterol, high LDL cholesterol, low HDL cholesterol, or elevated triglycerides? (A simple blood test can tell you how you stand.)

pitals and thus have used male subjects exclusively. For every woman who has participated in a heart disease study, thousands of men have been tested, so the treatment of women is generally based on what works for men, with little more than an educated guess as to how female physiology and hormones alter the equation.

Doctors are still more likely to diagnose chest pains and difficulty in breathing in a woman as an anxiety attack, not a heart attack, especially if the woman is under 50. Most disturbing of all, women die more frequently during coronary surgery than men do. This is not because we're weaker—in general women recover better from surgery than men—but rather because our heart disease is far less likely to be caught in the early stages. By the time a woman ends up in the operating room, she is apt to be older than the man down the hall receiving the same surgery and her disease is likely to be much further advanced. Moreover, women have smaller arteries and veins than men, so many bypass procedures, which were developed primarily for male patients, don't work as well on women.

The solution: Study after study has shown that estrogen has a protective effect on the heart, halving the risk of serious coronary disease. There are two kinds of cholesterol, the "bad" LDL, which carries fat to the blood vessel walls and thus causes blocked arteries, and the "good" HDL, which carries fat away from the blood vessel walls to the liver, where it is subsequently eliminated. Estrogen works to keep the level of HDL high, and if it is withdrawn, the percentage of LDL rises sharply. When lost estrogen is replaced, a healthy balance between HDL and LDL is restored.

Of course, simply going on HRT is not the only way you can lessen your chance of heart disease. You should also:

- Make sure that less than 30 percent of your daily caloric intake comes from fat.
- Hold your cholesterol intake to under 300 mg a day.
- Exercise aerobically at least three times a week.
- Avoid cigarette smoke.
- Stay within an appropriate weight range for your height and frame.

If you have a genetic history and/or lifestyle that predisposes you to coronary problems, or if you have a complicating condition such as diabetes or hypertension, you should educate yourself about what you can do to lower your risk. Making the lifestyle changes we recommend in chapter 6 is a good start, but if you have a serious family or personal history of heart disease, you and your doctor should discuss an individualized health-care program that includes close monitoring.

The bad news about heart disease is that it is rampant. More than half a million people die every year in the U.S. from heart attacks, and 50 percent of them are women. The good news is that we can do much to lower our personal risks, beginning with replacing the female hormones that give us such a coronary advantage in the years before menopause. This is one area in which equality with men is a big step backward for women.

Osteoporosis

The problem: The problem is that you don't know there is a problem. Osteoporosis frequently goes undiagnosed until the age of 70, when you fall and break a hip. Or, more likely, you break a hip and fall.

While a skipped period or night sweat is irritating, osteoporosis is long-term and debilitating. During perimenopause, a woman may lose 1 to 1.5 percent of her total bone mass each year. After menopause, the rate of bone loss accelerates to an average of 3 percent a year, with some women losing an astounding 6 percent a year. As the bones become thinner, they snap easily, resulting in breaks from the most minor actions, such as stepping off a curb. The back vertebrae, wrists, and hips are the most likely bones to break. Women in the advanced stages are capable of breaking bones by coughing or rolling over in bed.

There is a genetic link in osteoporosis, so if your mother or grandmother experienced bone breaks, became noticeably shorter as she aged, or developed the hump back that frequently comes with the disease, consider yourself at higher than average risk. In general, small, frail, fair-skinned white or Asian women are more prone to the disease than tall, big-boned, or black women.

Lifestyle choices can also raise your risk. If you have insufficient calcium in your diet, don't exercise, smoke, or have more than two alcoholic drinks a day, you've begun to undermine the strength of your skeletal system. A woman who enters perimenopause with lighter than average bones is the proverbial accident waiting to happen. Once the estrogen withdrawal of perimenopause begins, her risk doubles because she's not only prone to lose bone mass faster than a woman in better health but she has weaker bones to begin with.

Women who go through menopause before age 45, whether naturally or through surgery or chemotherapy, are also at increased risk, simply because they have fewer years in which to build up their bones and more years in which their bones are eroding.

How prevalent is osteoporosis? By age 60, 25 percent of white and Asian women will develop a spinal compression fracture, which is the gradual breaking down of the vertebrae of the spinal column, causing the bones literally to collapse upon each other. Women with this condition become shorter, develop the humpbacked look, and are on track for major spinal problems as they continue to age. Women lose an average of 2.5 inches in height between the age of menopause and age 80.

Other bone fractures follow. Femur and wrist fractures occur around age 70 and by the age of 80, 20 percent of American women will break a hip. Recovery from a hip fracture is slow, painful, and often incomplete, with a full 50 percent of hip-replacement patients never again able to live on their own. Heavy doses of pain medication are frequently required, sometimes causing the elderly women who are the most common victims of the disease to become permanently confused. It's hard to understand why more attention isn't paid to this largely avoidable disease, which causes so many women to end up experiencing chronic pain, using walkers, and living in nursing homes before their time.

The solution: Part of the reason osteoporosis isn't mentioned more often is that it's often asymptomatic until the moment a bone breaks. Since 25 percent of bone mass

---

Risk Factors for Osteoporosis

1. Are you Caucasian or Asian?
2. Did you experience menopause before age 45?
3. Do you have a family history of osteoporosis?
4. Are you thinner than average? Small boned?
5. Do you have or have you ever had low calcium intake?
6. Have you ever been anorexic? Did your periods ever stop for an extended length of time due to an eating disorder or excessive exercise?
7. Do you smoke?
8. Do you drink more than two glasses of an alcohol beverage per day?
9. Do you drink more than two beverages with caffeine daily?
10. Are you sedentary?
11. Do you take an anticonvulsant or glucocorticoid on a regular basis?
12. Do you suffer from any of the following medical conditions: menstrual irregularities, hyperthyroidism, Cushing's disease, chronic renal failure, or hypogonadism?

may be lost before it shows up on a routine X ray, most of the women who are in the early stages of osteoporosis don't know it.

As is dramatically illustrated in Figures 5.1 and 5.2, healthy bone is far heavier and denser than bone that has been ravaged by osteoporosis. Due to a variety of factors—skeletal type, a sedentary lifestyle, smoking and drinking, or a history of a low-calcium diet—a woman may arrive at perimenopause with lighter than average bones. If you have several of the risk factors listed on page 83, you should consider having your bones evaluated prior to menopause.

A dual energy X ray absorptiometry (DEXA) can better detect early bone loss than a standard X ray. Available at most hospitals and many clinics and satellite facilities, a DEXA is a relatively quick (3 to 5 minutes) low-dosage radiation technique, used to measure a woman's overall

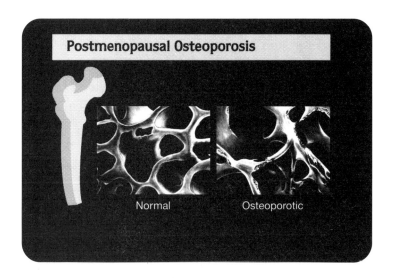

Figure 5.1 X ray of normal and osteoporotic bones.

bone density and to evaluate the lumbar spinal bones, which generally disintegrate first, and the femoral neck, the bone that breaks at the hip. A woman at high risk should have a DEXA around the age of 40 to serve as a baseline, like a baseline mammogram, against which to monitor future changes.

Once an accurate measurement of your bone density has been obtained prior to menopause, a follow-up DEXA can be done a year to 18 months after your last period. If there has been a significant decrease in bone density, you are at a high personal risk for osteoporosis. If this is the case, you should begin an aggressive preventative treatment—possibly HRT— immediately.

Considering how ravaging osteoporosis is, and how astronomical the costs of treatment are, why aren't DEXA tests done more frequently? DEXA is available at most

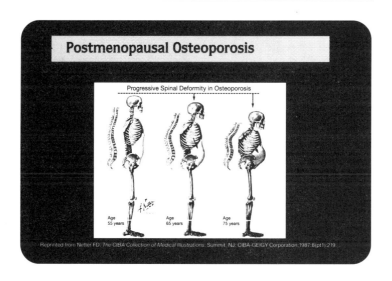

Figure 5.2 Skeletons of women with osteoporosis.

hospitals and medical centers. It costs about $200, but like most preventive medicine tools, it's ultimately cost-effective, especially when you consider that not only are surgery and physical therapy costly to both individuals and the public health-care system, but that half of all hip-replacement patients require nursing-home care for the rest of their lives.

Since women are the group most at risk for osteoporosis, this disease may be another example of women's health problems receiving more cavalier treatment than men's. Also, the victims of osteoporosis are largely elderly, and thus silent when it comes to lobbying the health-care system. But if we baby boomers live en masse into our 80s, as predicted, osteoporosis will be a major hurdle to maintaining our independence, and it's in our best interests to be vocal about this disease before we experience it. Since bone disease is largely preventable, and even in many cases reversible, at the very least we should demand that the major diagnostic test, the DEXA, be regularly recommended and covered by insurance. For more information, call or write the National Osteoporosis Foundation listed in the Sources section at the back of the book.

Building Better Bones Now

What can you do now to prevent osteoporosis in your own body? Start by developing dense bones prior to menopause. Calcium is essential for strong bones, and it is recommended that a menopausal woman at risk for osteoporosis take 1,500 mg daily. This is twice the normal recommended dosage and the equivalent of five 8-ounce glasses of milk a day, so you'll probably need supplements to meet the requirement. Large amounts of calcium are difficult to absorb at once, so it is better to take smaller doses at regular intervals, such as 500 mg before each meal. Vitamin D helps the body absorb calcium; 500 international units of vitamin D a day is standard. Magnesium and vitamin K also aid in bone repair. Vitamin K is present in so many foods, including almost all vegetables, that deficiency is rare, but 600 mg of magnesium daily will round out your bone-building program.

Both weight-bearing exercise (any activity, such as walking, where your body is forced to support its own weight) and weight-resistance exercise (such as Nautilus, working out with dumbbells or rubberized bands) build bone mass. A sedentary lifestyle sets you up for weaker bones that snap more easily. It is also important to stop smoking and limit your intake of both alcohol and coffee; nicotine, caffeine and alcohol all inhibit your body's ability to absorb calcium.

A woman whose DEXA reveals good bones and who has no familial predisposition toward osteoporosis may be able to prevent the disease through vitamin therapy, proper diet, exercise, and a health-conscious lifestyle. But if your DEXA indicates lighter than average bones or you have genetic risk factors, you'll need estrogen.

Hormone replacement therapy is a powerful weapon in the battle to maintain stronger bones because estrogen not only retards bone loss but in some cases actually seems to reverse osteoporosis by increasing bone density. HRT is not a quick-fix solution, however. When a woman stops HRT she will begin once again to lose bone mass at her previous rate. While the woman who merely has perimenopausal symptoms may be able to make do with a little transitional estrogen, the woman whose main goal in HRT is to prevent osteoporosis will have to continue the therapy even after her perimenopausal symptoms subside. Note: Some women opt for a lower dosage of estrogen after their symptoms abate. If you do, the nonhormonal methods of bone maintenance listed previously are a vital supplement to your HRT.

We spoke with one very active woman in her 40s who broke an ankle while playing volleyball with her young children. Her doctor was hesitant to use pins to set the fracture because the bones surrounding the break were so brittle he feared the process of inserting the pin would crack them. Concerned enough to have a follow-up DEXA, she learned that her bones were much lighter than average and began a vigorous program of osteoporosis prevention, as did her sister who, it turned out, had the same condition. Most women are not privy to information about their bones until it is far too late for preventive medicine, which is why a DEXA can be a helpful diagnostic tool if you suspect you may be at risk for bone disease.

Breast Cancer

The problem: HRT has been linked to a higher incidence of breast cancer, though the studies are either inconclusive or conflicting.

No other connection frightens women as much as this one. While osteoporosis and heart disease ultimately kill six times more women than cancer, most of those women are over the age of 60. Breast cancer is scary precisely because it can strike when a woman is young and seemingly healthy; one-third of the women who die from breast cancer are under 50, meaning you may well know a woman your age who has been diagnosed with the disease. Breast cancer looms large in the minds of many perimenopausal women as something that could happen to them, so they approach estrogen therapy with suspicion.

A link between breast cancer and HRT makes sense in theory. Women who start their periods earlier than normal or who go through a later than typical menopause have a higher risk of breast cancer, presumably because their bodies have been exposed to estrogen longer. Also, some breast tumors grow in response to estrogen, and many women who have breast cancer respond favorably to an estrogen-blocking medication called Tamoxifen.

These commonsense observations have been enough to prompt concern about the connection between estrogen and breast cancer, but the trouble is that three major studies have yielded three somewhat different results. Let's start with the depressing and indisputable fact that the average American woman has a 10 percent chance of contracting breast cancer in her lifetime, and then ask: If she takes HRT, what happens to that 10 percent risk?

1. The Center for Disease Control concluded that if a woman has been on HRT for 15 years, her risk rises by 30 percent. (Note: A 30 percent increase in a 10-percent base risk would raise a woman's personal chances of getting breast cancer to 13 percent, not 40 percent.) Women who were on estrogen for five years or less showed no increased risk.

2. A study done by Vanderbilt University found no increased risk among women taking estrogen in the standard 0.625 mg dose. Since many of the subjects of the Center for Disease Control study had been on estrogen for 15 years or longer, most began taking HRT in the high-dosage days of the 1970s. Consequently, some doctors argue that the Vanderbilt study is more relevant for women just beginning HRT.

3. Finally, the ongoing Nurses' Health Study conducted at Harvard University concluded that a woman who once took estrogen but stopped has no increased risk and that only women currently on estrogen bear the 30 percent higher risk. This means once you stop taking estrogen, your risk drops to its previous, lower level. The Nurses' Health Study also suggests that estrogen promotes

the growth of existing tumors rather than causing new tumors to develop. In other words, estrogen doesn't cause cancer, but it accelerates the growth of preexisting cancer cells. Because of the length of time the women were monitored and the large number (more than 100,000) included, the Nurses' Health Study is considered one of the most important studies ever conducted in the field of breast cancer.

What all three studies conclude in common is that short-term use of HRT doesn't significantly increase your risk of breast cancer; a woman has to be on estrogen for more than five years before her risk climbs. Since dosage also seems to affect breast cancer risk, some doctors advocate a 0.625 dose of estrogen while the woman is going through menopause and experiencing symptoms, followed by a smaller 0.3 dosage once she is past the age of 60 and requires less estrogen to suppress her symptoms.

Although women with personal risk factors working against them are considered to be at elevated risk, the disturbing truth is that it's extremely hard to predict who will get breast cancer. Eighty percent of the women diagnosed with the disease have no increased-risk factors at all. Questions about estrogen use keep resurfacing partly because we are still years away from understanding who is most likely to get breast cancer.

Advice for the Woman with a Family History of Breast Cancer

The Nurses' Health Study raises troubling issues for women with family histories of breast cancer or who have had the disease themselves. Since estrogen may accelerate the growth of existing tumors, is hormone therapy ever advisable for women at high risk for breast cancer?

Risk Factors for Breast Cancer

1. Did you begin having periods earlier than average (before the age of 12)?

2. Did you have a later than average menopause (after the age of 54)?

3. Were you over 30 when your first child was born?

4. Are you childless?

5. Are you obese?

6. Is your diet high in fat?

7. Do you have a mother or sister who has had breast cancer?

8. If you do have a close relative (mother or sister) with the disease, was she diagnosed before the age of 50?

9. Are you Caucasian? (Caucasian women living in the Western Hemisphere have the highest statistical rate of breast cancer in the world.)

Most doctors feel that it's safe to take estrogen on a short-term basis even if you have a family history of breast cancer. The majority of the doctors surveyed said they would not hesitate to prescribe transitional HRT for a couple of years for a woman who was experiencing disruptive symptoms.

Should you take HRT on a long-term basis if you have a mother or sister who has had breast cancer? This question is stickier. A woman with a first-degree family history of breast cancer has a 25 percent chance of developing the disease; if her relative risk rises by 30 percent with long-term HRT, her personal risk will be in the 31- to 33-percent range—frighteningly high. But does her relative risk rise by a full 30 percent? No one knows. The lone study done specifically on women who have family histories of breast cancer and who have taken long-term HRT showed that their risk rose only slightly, remaining around 25 percent, HRT or no HRT. But since only one study has been carried out and it used a relatively small number of subjects, HRT for these women remains a tough call to make.

The tiebreaker is how badly you need the therapy. If your risk for heart disease or osteoporosis equals or exceeds your risk for breast cancer, long-term HRT may still be your best choice.

Advice for the Woman with a Personal History of Breast Cancer

The Nurses' Health Study showed that, although estrogen doesn't appear to cause breast cancer, it may reactivate residual cancer in women who have previously had the disease. Most doctors are reluctant to prescribe HRT for women who have had cancer, but even this rule is open to debate. One recent study examined the use of HRT for six months in women who had previously had breast cancer. It showed that after two years no cases of tumor reactivation were found. (Note that this is very short-term use of HRT.)

At present, this decision should be analyzed on a case-by-case basis. A physician will probably consider three factors:

> 1. How long has the woman been cancer-free? Many doctors offer HRT to women who have had no cancer for five or more years, arguing that there is no evidence that estrogen aggravates successfully treated cancer. Other doctors contend that there's no evidence that it doesn't aggravate dormant cancer and that—considering women who have

had breast cancer bear a sixfold greater than normal risk of redeveloping the disease—it would be foolish to take even the slightest chance.

2. How badly is the patient suffering? Short-term use for a patient with debilitating symptoms might be recommended.

   Also, if a woman is already in the final stages of cancer and is suffering from severe estrogen-deficiency symptoms, her physician may prescribe HRT in an effort to improve the quality of the months or years she has left.

3. What is the patient's risk for heart disease and osteoporosis? Long-term use for a patient with no particular risk would probably not be recommended. Some doctors will prescribe HRT for former cancer patients if they have a particularly high risk of heart disease or are already showing signs of rapid bone loss.

Tamoxifen

A drug that blocks the effects of estrogen, tamoxifen is frequently prescribed for women with breast cancer because it prevents the growth of malignant cells. Strangely enough, this anti-estrogen drug acts like estrogen in the body, offering some protection against osteoporosis and heart disease.

Tamoxifen doesn't help hot flashes, vaginal dryness, and the other transitional symptoms of perimenopause, and 5 percent of the women who take it report side effects such as nausea and bloating. But for a women who has had breast cancer, a drug that opposes malignant cells while protecting her bones and heart can seem like a godsend. Tamoxifen may be a valid option for many women who can't take HRT.

Cancer Screening

The monthly self-exam is your first line of defense against breast cancer. Designate a certain time each month to do the exam—after your period, if you're still having them, or when you pay the electric bill, if you're not—and if you have any doubts about the effectiveness of your technique, ask your doctor or nurse to show you how. An annual check by a medical professional is an added safety net.

We all know the importance of having mammograms, but there are several schools of thought on how often we should have them. The American Cancer Society recommends a baseline mammogram by age 35 or before beginning HRT; after that, some physicians recommend annual mammograms while others say that such frequency subjects you to unnecessary radiation and that every two years will suffice. Talk to your doctor. Your personal risk factors may make the difference as to how often he or she advises a mammogram.

A final note: Some women report that their doctors started them on hormone therapy with no discussion of breast cancer at all. If your physician prescribes HRT without discussing your personal breast cancer risk and screening techniques, that's a flashing neon sign that this person is not equipped to help you manage your perimenopause.

Facts to Keep in Mind

1. Heart disease kills more than half of the women in the U.S. over 50, and osteoporosis affects one-quarter of white American women. Your odds of getting one of these diseases significantly outweighs the 10 percent chance you'll contract breast cancer. This is the reason most doctors feel the benefits of HRT make it worth the risks.

2. The scary studies about long-term use of HRT were done primarily on women who took estrogen during the high-dosage days of the 1970s. Until enough years have passed that studies can be done on women who have spent a decade on the lower-dosage pills, we can't say with certainty that lower doses translate into lower risks, but it seems logical that they would.

3. Short-term use of HRT appears to have no effect on a woman's chances of contracting cancer, so if you would like HRT to ease you through the transitions of perimenopause, there is no reason not to take it.

4. Even in a worst-case scenario, long-term use of HRT makes a woman's risk rise by 30 percent, raising her personal risk of contracting breast cancer in her lifetime to 13 percent. None of this is to belittle the very real fears women have about breast cancer; a 13 percent chance is still far too high, and if you're one of the women who contracts cancer, all the stats about heart disease are going to be of precious little comfort to you. Just be aware that the increase in breast cancer risk that accompanies long-term HRT is not as high as you may have thought.

5. Many doctors conclude that estrogen does not increase a healthy woman's chance of getting breast cancer. They argue that estrogen is a natural substance, produced by the body for more than 40 years, and that replacing it after it's lost won't "give" you cancer. However, if tumors are already present, estrogen speeds their growth, making the long-term use of HRT risky for women who have previously had cancer and for women who have such high-risk factors that they may have malignancies of which they're currently unaware.

The Bottom Line

One of the reasons that we're all so frightened about this issue is we've talked ourselves into believing that any decision we make is irreversible. It's as if we're standing at a fork in the road with breast cancer lurking in one direction and a heart attack in the other.

It's key to remember that the risk of cancer for ever-users and never-users is identical. Once you stop taking HRT, your risks, for good or for ill, revert back to their previous levels. This means that HRT is not a once-in-a-lifetime decision, but rather a year-by-year decision that can be altered anytime. You may start on HRT, have a scary mammogram, and conclude that it isn't worth it.

Condition	Mortality Age 50–75 per 100,000
Heart Disease	10,500
Breast Cancer	1,875
Osteoporotic Fractures	938
Endometrial Cancer	188
Gallbladder Disease	3

Death rate per 100,000 women aged 50 to 75 from diseases affected, positively or negatively, by estrogen. Approximately five times as many women die each year of heart disease than breast cancer. Almost half as many women die of osteoporotic fractures (primarily hip) as die of breast cancer. Endometrial cancer is a negligible risk if progestin is added to estrogen replacement.

(derived from Henderson *et al*, American Journal Obstet Gynecol 154:1181, 1986)

Figure 5.3 Relative Risks of Conditions Affected by Estrogen.

You may vow, "No HRT for me," learn through a DEXA three years later that you're losing bone mass rapidly and be forced to reconsider.

The bottom line on all this risky business? Assess your personal risks for heart disease, osteoporosis, and breast cancer, as well as your present level of perimenopausal discomfort (see Figure 5.3 and Figure 5.4). Then, if you decide you need HRT, go ahead. We already know that the risk for short-term use is minimal, and by the time you move from short-term to long-term use, studies should be released with information based on the new,

Condition	Risk	*Changes in Mortality Age 50–75 per 100,000*
Heart Disease	0.5 RR	–5.250
Osteoporotic Fractures	0.4 RR	–5.63
Endometrial Cancer	2.0 RR	+6.3
Gallbladder Disease	1.5 RR	+2

For women taking estrogen, change in relative risk (RR) of dying from conditions influenced by estrogen. A woman on estrogen has a 50 percent risk of dying from heart disease compared to a woman not on estrogen. Estrogen reduces the chance of dying from an osteoporotic fracture to 40 percent of that of a woman not on estrogen. The RR of a woman dying from endometrial cancer is doubled if she is on estrogen, but this is only if she is on unopposed estrogen (i.e., without progestin).

(derived from Henderson *et al*, American Journal Obstet Gynecol 154:1181, 1986)

Figure 5.4 Estimated Mortality Changes Induced by Estrogen.

lower dosages. On the other hand, if your complaints are minor, your bones and heart test out healthy, and you don't need HRT, don't take it. Either way, view the decision as a temporary one.

Then reassess. Reassess with each new mammogram, DEXA or cholesterol test, each new symptom, and each new study. Medicine can be introduced or removed from your system as circumstances dictate. Estrogen does not linger in the body for years. If it did, we wouldn't go through menopause in the first place.

6

Wellness, Part One:
Diet, Exercise,
and Nutrition

Health is more than the absence of disease. Ideally, we strive for wellness, a state of feeling energetic, alert, and in charge of our bodies and our lives. If you think of your health care as simply solving problems as they develop, you're taking the passive, or reactive, approach. Wellness requires "pro-action"—heading off pain and disease before they occur and focusing not just on the isolated symptom but on the bigger issues of relaxation, balance, movement, and nutrition.

If you have thought about making changes—exercising more, eating better, giving up coffee or cigarettes—perimenopause is the perfect time to put those good intentions into action. A short-term problem, such as insomnia or a sudden weight gain, may initially prompt you, but the changes you make now will have long-term consequences, helping to determine not only how long you live, but how well you live.

Weight Control

Are we doomed to gain weight during the menopausal years? Most women do, and those who are already obese gain more than women who enter menopause at a normal weight. Women on average gain 10 to 15 pounds after menopause; obese women gain an average of 21 to 23 pounds.

In many cases, the weight gain can be traced to a lower metabolic rate. After menopause, your lean body mass begins to decrease while your fat body mass begins to increase. Fat is inert, and your body doesn't have to work hard to sustain it. So the fatter you become, the less fuel your body requires. Do we sense a cycle starting here? Since a stalled metabolism means you're burning fewer calories, you can gain weight even if you're eating the same amount you've eaten for years.

This is precisely why so many women are frustrated by their mid-life weight gain. They argue that they aren't overeating, and if you define overeating as eating more than in years past, they aren't. But if an inactive lifestyle and lack of muscle mass have combined to slow your metabolic rate, you can gain weight on 1,800 calories a day—which hardly anyone in our culture would consider overeating. By taking in only 200 more calories each day than you expend, you will gain approximately 20 pounds in a year.

Do Hormones Affect Weight Gain?

Taking HRT doesn't seem to have an effect on whether or not you gain weight. A recent HRT versus no-HRT study showed similar weight gains in the hormone-treated and control groups. However, hormones may affect where you carry the weight.

The fat postmenopausal women accumulate tends to cluster around their abdomens in the "apple" distribution associated more with men and an increased risk of heart disease. Prior to menopause, most women who are over-weight have a gynecoid distribution, that is, a "pear" body type, with their fat mainly on their hips and thighs. Since women tend to start out pear-shaped and become more apple-shaped after menopause, it makes sense that this new fat distribution pattern may be due to hormonal changes.

Studies are inconclusive but have suggested that HRT reverses the menopausal tendency toward apple distribution, encouraging future fat to maintain the pear distribution. This is not simply a cosmetic debate: fat in the abdominal area is far more dangerous to the heart than fat in the hip and thigh area.

How Fat Is Fat?

DEXA, the test that measures bone density, can also be used to measure body fat percentage. Submersion tests, based on a long-known fact that fat floats and lean body mass sinks, is another accurate way of calculating how much fat you're carrying. If you can't travel to a hospital or full-scale spa for a DEXA or submersion test, at least ask your doctor or gym to give you a caliper skin test. A device that measures surface fat by lightly pinching the skin on the arm and hip, a caliper can give you a basic idea of where you stand.

How much of your body is fat is vital information, for a scale tells only half of the story. Weight doesn't affect our long-term health as much as percentage of fat. Some thin-looking but sedentary women have more fat than the desirable 18-to-25-percent range, and, conversely, some active women weigh more than you might think. This was dramatically proven to us when an aerobics instructor, who had a body every woman in her class admired, climbed on the spa scales to prove she weighed 145 pounds. Anyone would have guessed she was 20 pounds lighter, but this was a woman with very toned muscles, and muscle, while weighing more than fat, takes up less room. At 145 pounds, she had an enviably low body fat percentage of 15 percent.

Muscle Mass: The Missing Component in Weight Loss

The vast majority of us are not professional athletes, nor do we necessarily aspire to vein-bulging muscles. But any woman can increase her muscle mass to the point where her metabolism is higher. Obviously, exercise burns fat while you are exercising, but, by forcing the body to work harder to maintain its newer, hungrier muscles, exercise also helps you to burn fat even while resting.

Adults on average lose a half pound of muscle mass every year after age 20; in women over 35, the rate of loss accelerates to one pound a year. With each lost pound of muscle, you burn 50 fewer calories a day. Happily, the formula also works in reverse. With each pound of muscle you develop, your body will require 50 additional calories a day, meaning that if an active 130-pound woman has five more pounds of muscle than an inactive 130-pound woman, the active woman can eat 250 more calories a day than the inactive woman. If the inactive woman took in the same caloric amount as the active woman, she would gain more than 20 pounds in the course of a single year.

For this reason, an increased activity level is more vital than diet to the menopausal woman who is fighting obesity. If your food intake hasn't increased but your weight has, don't try eating less. Try moving more.

Exercise

The advantages to regular physical activity are numerous and well-documented. Exercise:

♦ maintains bone density, especially if you choose a weight-bearing exercise.

♦ maintains muscle mass.

♦ increases metabolism, burning calories and fat.

♦ reduces the risks of cancer, diabetes, and heart disease.

♦ reduces stress.

♦ alleviates many symptoms of menopause (including some you might not guess, such as hot flashes).

♦ helps former smokers stay off cigarettes.

♦ may affect the immune system, making you less vulnerable to communicable diseases such as colds and flu.

♦ helps maintain flexibility and joint movement as we age.

Types of Exercise

The three basic types of exercise are aerobics, weight resistance, and flexibility training.

Aerobic Exercise The most vital kind of exercise, this category includes walking, running, swimming, biking, and aerobic dance. The primary function of aerobics is to burn fat and work the heart and lungs. If the aerobic exercise is weight-bearing (the body is upright and supports its own weight), then the activity also increases your bone and muscle strength. Among these activities are walking, running, dance, using a cross-country ski machine, and bench stepping.

For women with arthritis or a history of joint injuries, weight-bearing exercise is probably not an option. Swimming is an excellent cardiovascular workout, and a water aerobics class is another good choice, since a well-run class will not only challenge you aerobically but also provide some resistance and flexibility work.

Aerobic activity three times a week will protect the heart, but to build strength effectively, aerobics should be done five to seven days per week for at least 30 minutes at a time. If weight loss is a primary goal, increase your time, not your intensity: exercise for 45 to 60 minutes a day, five to seven days a week.

Weight Resistance   This doesn't have to mean an hour on the Nautilus machines, although you might enjoy this more than you would guess. You can maintain muscle mass with light, hand-held weights or the special rubber bands that create resistance. To work the abdominal muscles, crunches should be part of your weight-resistance routine.

Many women skip this important step in fitness, arguing that they don't want a muscle-bound look. In truth, very few women have enough testosterone in their systems to produce huge muscles. The goal of weight resistance is simply to create a well-toned, tight look.

If you want to build muscle mass, not merely maintain it, join a gym. A serious weight program should be followed under the supervision of an instructor or personal trainer. Three weekly sessions are recommended, so that all the major muscle groups are worked in the course of a week. Weight training also builds stronger bones, especially in the upper body, which is often neglected in aerobic exercise.

Flexibility   The component most likely to be ignored, this type of exercise is especially important for women as they age. Many kinds of flexibility work, such as yoga, t'ai chi, ballet, and simple stretching, have the added bonus of reducing stress and improving sleep.

Remember when bananas were being touted as the ideal food? Actually, no one food can give you everything you need, nor can one exercise, but walking is the closest thing we have to a banana in the exercise world. A 30-minute walk will provide aerobic benefits with minimal expense and chance of injury. Gradually increase your pace and your duration.

For an exercise program to last, however, you'll need to forestall boredom and burnout. Women who incorporate more than one type of activity into their exercise programs—they swim three days a week and walk three, for example, or they join a gym that offers a variety of classes—stay with it longer than those who grimly follow the same routine every day.

If you're walking, varying your route can reduce boredom, and some women listen to books or music on headsets, which is especially good if you walk on a track or treadmill and don't have to stay alert to traffic. "It's my think time," says a woman who has walked her way through the *New York Times* best-seller list, three miles at a clip. Finding an exercise partner can also hold you to it, either because you know a friend is waiting to walk with you on your lunch hour or because the gym becomes not only a place to work out, but also your social time. Seeing friends on a regular basis is good for the heart too.

Frequency and Intensity of Exercise

Your target heart-rate range is an internal speedometer: it tells you exactly how fast you should go. Just as it's dangerous to drive 70 miles per hour in a 45 zone, it's foolish and unnecessary to exceed your body's natural limit by exercising too hard.

You can find your target range using the following formula:

1. Measure your resting pulse (heart rate).

    ____a____ beats per minute

2. Subtract your age from 220 to determine your predicted maximum heart rate.

    $220 - $ ___age___ $= $ ___b___

3. Subtract your resting heart rate from your predicted maximum heart rate.

    ____b____ $-$ ___a___ $=$ ___c___

4. Multiply ___c___ by 60 percent and by 85 percent.

___c___	___c___
$\times\ .60$	$\times\ .85$
d_1	d_2

5. Add your resting heart rate to d_1 and d_2.

    ____d_1____ $+$ ___a___ $=$ _____

    ____d_2____ $+$ ___a___ $=$ _____

    These two numbers represent the lower and upper limits of your target heart-rate range.

Using this formula, a moderately fit 40-year-old woman may find her target training heart rate to be between 110 and 150 beats per minute. Exercising for 20 to 30 minutes within that range will bring her cardiovascular benefits. If weight loss is a goal, she should exercise longer, not harder, keeping her heart rate in the lower end of her training range. An hour of brisk walking with a heart rate of 120 will burn more fat than 20 minutes of high-intensity aerobics with a heart rate of 150.

Note: If your resting heart rate is unusually low or unusually high (lower than 55 or higher than 90), check with your physician before beginning an exercise program.

The Perfect One-Hour Workout

Warm-up   Start with 10 minutes of gentle exercise to warm up. Whatever activity you have chosen, begin slowly and gradually pick up speed, moving into your target heart range toward the end of the warm-up period. The easiest way to tell when you're moving into your target range is to have a watch or clock nearby with a visible second hand. Put two fingertips to your throat just below your jaw and find your pulse, then count your heartbeats for six seconds. Let's say you feel 12 beats. If you add a zero to this number, you are in effect multiplying a six-second count by 10 and estimating how many times your heart is beating in a minute. Your count of 12 indicates a heart rate of about 120, which means that you're moving into the aerobic phase of your workout.

Target Range   Maintain the activity for 20 to 30 minutes, working within your target heart range. Do the pulse check twice during the course of your workout to make sure your heart rate isn't too high. If it is, don't stop abruptly, just slow your pace until your heart rate recovers to a resting range.

Another way to monitor your training level is the "perceived exertion" method, which is a fancy way of saying that if you feel like you're getting ready to pass out, you probably are. In your ideal training range, you should feel like you're working fairly hard and, as one exercise instructor put it, still be able to talk but not quite able to sing. If you are gasping, or feel dizzy, ease up.

Cool-down   Continue the activity for five more minutes at a slower pace until you are back to the level of exertion you experienced during your warm-up.

Stretching   Take five minutes to stretch out. Your high school PE teacher may have advocated stretching before exercise, but we now know that overextending a cold muscle is asking for injury. Save your stretches for the end of the aerobic phase, when your muscles are warm.

Weight Training   Use the final 10 minutes of the hour to work with light weights or rubber resistance bands, or to do modified push-ups and abdominal crunches. Since you don't want to work the same muscle groups two days in a row, you might opt to do upper body one day, lower body the next. The abdominals, we regret to inform you, can be safely exercised every day.

Some Commonsense Precautions

1. If you're over the age of 35 and have health-risk factors or have been extremely inactive, see your doctor before starting an exercise progam. If you're over 50 when beginning, you should definitely see your doctor and request an evaluation to determine your precise target heart rate.

2. Exercise must be regular. If you're not going to do even 20 minutes three times a week, don't bother working out at all. A weekend exercise blitz—when a sedentary person plays three straight hours of tennis—is more dangerous than helpful.

3. Stop if you feel short of breath, a strained muscle, joint pain, or numbness and tingling, especially in the chest or arms.

4. Use the right shoes. Exercise has become shoe-specific, with walking shoes available for walking,

step shoes for step aerobics, and countless running and aerobic dance shoes. At $60 a pop for a good pair of workout shoes, you may be tempted to use one pair for every activity, but don't. An investment in proper shoes is far cheaper than a trip to an orthopedic surgeon.

5. Should you exercise when you feel sick? Use the "neck check" to decide. If your ailment is above the neck—a headache, stuffy nose, or sneezing—try exercising for 10 minutes and then evaluate how you feel. If you feel fine, continue. But if your complaint is below the neck—a bad chest cough, stomach pain, or muscle strain—skip a day or two.

6. Drink eight ounces of water before and after exercising. Don't rely on thirst as an indicator of how much water you need.

7. If the temperature plus humidity equals 150 or higher, exercise indoors.

8. Most important, if you need instruction, get it. Your local YMCA or community college probably sponsors aerobics classes, running clinics, even tips on walking and biking. It is essential to receive instruction on weight training and flexibility exercises. Books or exercise tapes can give you ideas about how to get started, but if you plan to go past the basics, take a class and ask the instructor to check your technique while lifting or stretching.

Diet

As kids we learned about "the four food groups," a dietary system that pronounced all types of food to be equally important to a "balanced" diet. Today the four groups have been replaced by the food pyramid, a system that suggests we eat plenty of complex carbohydrates, which form the wide base of the pyramid, and very little of the fats and oils that make up the top. The problem for most of us is that our dietary pyramids are so top-heavy they're ready to crumble.

Understanding the Dietary Pyramid

Let's work our way down the pyramid shown in Figures 6.1a and 6.1b. You're undoubtedly getting enough fat in your diet, and probably enough dairy and animal protein too. Most Americans eat two to three times the amount of protein recommended. But we don't eat enough of the foods that form the bottom of the pyramid—fruits, vegetables, and complex carbohydrates such as bread, pasta, cereal, and rice. A recent study indicated that the average American eats one vegetable a day.

The irony is that you can eat large amounts of the foods at the base of the pyramid without putting on weight, but eating too much of the calorie-dense foods at the top of the pyramid sets you up for weight gain. As a nation, we're eating too little of the foods we can and should consume quite freely, and way too much of the foods we should limit.

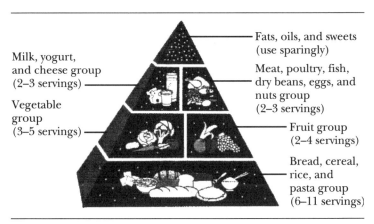

Figure 6.1a Food Pyramid

How to Use the Daily Food Guide

What counts as one serving?

Bread, Cereal, Rice, and Pasta
1 slice of bread
$^1/_2$ cup of cooked rice or pasta
$^1/_2$ cup of cooked cereal
1 ounce of ready-to-eat cereal

Vegetables
$^1/_2$ cup of chopped raw or cooked vegetables
1 cup of leafy raw vegetables

Fruit
1 whole fruit or melon wedge
$^3/_4$ cup of juice
$^1/_2$ cup of canned fruit
$^1/_4$ cup of dried fruit

Milk, Yogurt, and Cheese
1 cup of milk or yogurt
$1^1/_2$ to 2 ounces of cheese

Meat, Poultry, Fish, Dry Beans, Eggs, and Nuts
$2^1/_2$ to 3 ounces of cooked lean meat, poultry, or fish
Count $^1/_2$ cup of cooked beans or 1 egg or 2 tablespoons of peanut butter as 1 ounce of lean meat (about $^1/_3$ serving).

Fats, Oils, and Sweets
LIMIT CALORIES FROM THESE, especially if you need to lose weight.

How many servings do you need each day?

	Women & some older adults	Children, teen girls, active women, & most men	Teen boys & active men
Calorie level*	about 1,600	about 2,200	about 2,800
Bread group	6	9	11
Vegetable group	3	4	5
Fruit group	2	3	4
Milk group**	2–3	2–3	2–3
Meat group	2, for a total of 5 ounces	2, for a total of 6 ounces	3, for a total of 7 ounces

*These are the calorie levels if you choose lowfat, lean foods from the 5 major food groups and use foods from the fats, oils, and sweets group sparingly.

**Women who are pregnant or breast-feeding, teenagers, and young adults to age 24 need 3 servings.

Figure 6.1b How to interpret the food pyramid.

Dairy foods, nuts, and animal proteins are calorie-dense because of their high fat content. One gram of fat has nine calories, so you take in lots of calories, even through a small amount of food. Pure fats—oils, butter, mayonnaise, and salad dressings—are obvious trouble for people trying to watch their weight, but, unless defatted, dairy products are also apt to derive most of their caloric content from fat, not protein.

Protein has four calories per gram, so pure protein is not terribly dense in calories. Unfortunately, our protein rarely comes to us straight. Beef is marbled with fat, chicken is served with the skin left on, fish is deep-fried. Lean proteins, such as fish, shellfish, plainly cooked chicken, and fat-trimmed red meat, are fine in moderate amounts.

One gram of carbohydrate also has four calories, meaning you can eat a lot of food and still lose weight if you choose from the bottom of the pyramid. But Americans have trouble figuring what constitutes "a lot." It's safe to say that what you consider a serving size and what the dietitians who create the food charts consider a serving size are not the same thing. Remember, these are the people who claim you can feed a family of eight with one box of spaghetti.

Portion Size

Looking at the grains, a serving size is one slice of bread, $1/2$ cup of cooked rice or pasta, or one ounce of cereal. When you pour a bowl of cereal, you're more likely eating three ounces, and $1/2$ cup of pasta fills a saucer, not a plate. So while eight servings of grains may seem like an impossible goal, it actually translates into a bowl of cereal for breakfast, a sandwich at lunch, and spaghetti for dinner.

Misunderstanding serving size is only a mild problem when you're talking carbohydrates; the bigger problem is overeating in the dairy, animal protein, and fat categories. Take the time to measure out 3 ounces of meat or 1.5 ounces of cheese. To help you visualize, 4 ounces of meat is about the size of a deck of cards, and the average recommended amount for women is 5 to 6 ounces a day.

Inactive or older women require around 1,600 calories each day—while active women can eat up to 2,200 without gaining weight. If you're moderately active, just starting an exercise program, you can maintain your weight on 1,800 calories a day. This translates to 7 to 8 servings from the bread group, 3 from the fruit group, 3 to 4 from the vegetable group, 2 from the milk group, and 2 from the meat group for a total of 6 ounces. If you wish to lose weight, you should increase your exercise level, cut fats to a minimum, make sure all dairy products are skim, and decrease your meat to one serving a day. Keep your fruit, vegetable, and bread intake high.

Make Changes Gradually . . . and Permanently

Don't try to make all the changes at once. Gradually work lowfat eating into your lifestyle and increase exercise duration and intensity over time, so that you'll stick with it. Quick weight loss invariably leads to quick weight gain, so aim to lose no more than a pound a week. Such dramatic pledges as "I'll hold to 10 fat grams a day" or "I'll never eat fast food again" lead to dramatic lapses. Don't consider this a diet that you are either on or off; yo-yo dieting is stressful for the body and sets you up to regain more fat than you lost. Try instead to look at these as permanent changes: eating less fat instead of no fat, going out for two lunches a week and brown-bagging the rest, choosing the Ben & Jerry's Cherry Garcia frozen yogurt over the Cherry Garcia ice cream. This food plan is designed to help you feel better, not as punishment for all past sins.

Even with realistic goals, you may still hit the dreaded plateaus. If you're holding to your food plan without continuing to lose weight, don't give in to the temptation to cut your calorie intake drastically. A diet of fewer than 1,200 calories a day makes it nearly impossible to meet your nutritional needs and also causes your body to readjust its metabolism. Our bodies are naturally self-defensive, and if your body thinks it's starving, it will go on metabolic cruise control, burning fewer calories. A far better response to a plateau is to increase your exercise time, perhaps walking both in the morning and the evening, while keeping your food intake steady.

Nutrition

Nutrition sounds complicated, but there are three basic rules that, if followed, will go a long way in cutting your risk of disease:

1. Increase the level of antioxidants and phyto-chemicals in your body by eating more fruits and vegetables.
2. Cut back on fat.
3. Increase your fiber intake.

Let's look at each in detail.

Step One: Increase Your Antioxidants

Antioxidants are vitamins A, C, and E, and have been linked to decreased risks of cancer and heart disease. During oxidation, the body burns fuel and toxic substances called free radicals are released. Antioxidants pick up the free radicals before they can enter the organs and help the body excrete them.

Antioxidants have gotten tremendous amounts of press recently, and there is even some speculation that they are especially beneficial for people who live in an urban environment and are exposed to pollution. But while we wait for studies to conclude just how much good antioxidants can do, it's beyond dispute that they do good, and that the American diet is woefully deficient in the foods that contain them: green and yellow vegetables, citrus fruits, and wheat.

The Alliance for Aging Research recommends daily amounts of antioxidants that are up to four times higher than the current Recommended Daily Allowances set by the FDA.

FDA	*Alliance for Aging Research*
Vitamin A: 10 mg	Vitamin A: 30 mg
Vitamin C: 250 mgs	Vitamin C: 1000 mg
Vitamin E: 100 IU	Vitamin E: 400 IU

Unless you are already taking vitamin supplements or are unusually health-conscious, you're probably falling short of even the minimum requirements. It's often said that adults should receive all the recommended daily amounts of vitamins and minerals through a healthy diet, but probably no more than 25 percent of them do. You know yourself. If you're more inclined to hit the drive-through than pack a salad for lunch, face the facts and start taking vitamin and mineral supplements. Aim for dosages between the higher and lower recommendations. Anything the body doesn't need, it will excrete, leading to rather expensive urine—but better that than courting a health problem that could be avoided through such a simple preventive measure as taking a multivitamin.

Daily requirements of various vitamins and minerals—and the foods that are rich in them—are discussed below.

Vitamin A/Beta Carotene   This antioxidant is primarily found in the following green, leafy vegetables, yellow vegetables, and yellow fruits: carrots, spinach, squash, broccoli, lettuce, peaches, apricots, and sweet potatoes.

Your daily beta carotene needs can be met with two to three cups of these vegetables or fruits or with a 30 mg supplement.

Vitamin C   Disparate opinions as to the optimal daily quantity of this antioxidant range from 250 to 1,000 mg. Vitamin C is found in tomatoes, citrus fruits, (oranges, grapefruits, tangerines, lemons, pineapples, limes), broccoli, peppers, celery, cauliflower, kiwi fruit, and cantaloupe.

If you're not consuming two fruits or glasses of juice a day plus at least one vegetable from the list, consider taking a 500 mg supplement.

Vitamin E   Another antioxidant, and one with the added benefit of eliminating bad cholesterol (LDL), vitamin E is found in bran, wheat, nuts, and seeds (Note: These last two should be eaten sparingly because of their high fat content.)

If your diet is low in whole grains, supplement with 100 to 400 international units of vitamin E per day.

Phytochemicals   Phytochemicals are substances found in fruits and vegetables that researchers believe may have cancer-fighting properties. Since they are natural antioxidants, phytochemicals have a detoxifying effect, helping the body to eliminate harmful substances more efficiently. If you have a family history of cancer or if you smoke, drink considerable amounts of alcohol or caffeine, or live in a polluted environment, it makes sense to up your intake of phytochemicals, either by eating more fruits and vegetables or by taking antioxidant vitamin supplements.

Calcium   The importance of calcium in preventing osteoporosis is outlined in chapter 5. Between 1,000 and 1,500 mg daily is the recommendation for women over 35.

But calcium is tricky. It's not enough simply to get it into the body, there's also the problem of keeping it there. Certain drugs, such as tetracycline antibiotics, cholestyramine, and even Metamucil, can interfere with calcium absorption. A high intake of caffeine, nicotine, alcohol, or the phosphorus found in many processed foods and soft drinks can cause a woman to excrete calcium in her urine. Excessive protein, which is defined as more than 40 grams a day (not an unusual amount in this society), can also cause calcium deficiency and, ultimately, osteoporosis.

If you're concerned about maintaining calcium, limit your consumption of processed foods, protein, and caffeine. Soft drinks, which have both caffeine and phosphorus, are especially calcium-depleting. Cut out smoking and limit alcohol to two drinks a day or less. Taking 400 IU of vitamin D daily will also aid in calcium absorption.

Vitamin B-6   It has long been suspected that B-6 may function as a natural diuretic and thus ease PMS and perimenopausal symptoms, although this has not been proven. Taking it can't hurt, as long as you are careful not to exceed 25 mg a day. Too much B-6 can cause tingling or burning sensations on the skin.

Iron   Nutritionists used to advise iron supplements for almost all women since it was believed that the very process of menstruation depleted iron. But ionized iron is now known to be an oxidant, one of the bad boys associated with increased cancer risk and heart disease. So back off from the iron supplements; you're probably getting all you need through your diet, and megadoses of this mineral are unwise.

Step Two: Cut Fat

In the typical American diet, 37 percent of daily calories come from fat. Ideally, less than 30 percent of your calories should come from fat, and if you're trying to lose weight, the figure should be closer to 20 percent. The following suggestions will help you to reduce your fat intake.

1. Eat less visible fat. Either limit your use of all fat products, such as butter, oils, and salad dressings, or switch to the lowfat or nonfat varieties.

2. Eat less meat. Think of meat as a supplement, not as a major food group. One small chicken breast or a single hamburger patty is enough to satisfy an adult's daily protein requirement, but many people have trouble getting used to that idea. How do you cut down on meat when so many of our meals revolve around a "main course" of steak or chicken?

   Begin with meatless lunches; choose soup, salad, vegetarian chili, or meat-free pizza. Try to have one meatless dinner a week. On the other nights, select low-meat meals such as soups, stews, stir-frys, defatted casseroles, or salads with tuna or sliced chicken on top. When you're eating out, order a simply prepared meat such as broiled fish or opt for a cuisine like Japanese or Italian. A meal that consists primarily of rice or pasta, using meat as an accent, can make four ounces of protein seem like more.

3. Use lowfat or nonfat dairy products. The dairy industry has come a long way, offering a wider variety of lowfat cheeses, yogurts, sour creams, cottage cheeses, and imitation ice creams. Buy the new products in small amounts so you can taste-test them; some will probably strike you as rubbery or bland, but others may be close in flavor to the original.

Choose cheeses with fewer than five grams of fat per serving. If you're used to whole milk, gradually work your way down from 2 percent to 1 percent to $^1/_2$ percent to skim. Reconcile yourself slowly to the other fat-free products as well, perhaps mixing nonfat sour cream with whole sour cream on your baked potato or combining fat-free and standard cheeses in your lasagna until you adjust to the differences in taste and texture.

4. Read labels. Thanks to the Nutritional Labeling and Education Act of 1990, nutritional information on labels is much more complete than it used to be.

   Nonetheless, manufacturers can still mislead you. "Cholesterol-free" doesn't mean fat-free, and many products that proudly claim to have no cholesterol are loaded with fat. Another trick is basing calorie and fat estimates on a ridiculously small serving size. Does anyone really split a pint of frozen yogurt among six people?

   A good rule of thumb when looking at a label is to see whether there are more than two to three grams of fat per 100 calories. At three fat grams per 100 calories, you're bringing in your fat percentage at 30 percent. If you want to lose weight, you'll need to take it down to 20 percent, or two fat grams per 100 calories.

5. Educate yourself. Innumerable books on lowfat cooking are available, as are charts that allow you to calculate your fat intake down to the very last gram. Many hospitals and schools have economically priced or free classes on how to cook more healthfully, how to shop for lowfat foods, and how to read labels.

6. How you cook is as important as what you cook. Trim visible fat, including poultry skins, before cooking; otherwise the fat is absorbed into the meat during the cooking process.

Lowfat preparation techniques include steaming, poaching, boiling, broiling, baking, grilling, and microwaving. Marinating in fat-free dressing or blackening fish and chicken prior to cooking can add flavor without adding fat. Avoid frying or baking with added sauces or creams. In general, the more plain the food, the more likely it is to be low in fat.

A cookbook or class on lowfat cooking will give you ideas on how to grill seafood, stir-fry without oil or cut the amount of fat called for in a baked recipe.

7. Avoid fast food. Most chains now have a nutritional analysis available upon request, so if you eat fast food on a regular basis, ask to see the chart and study the fat contents of various items; there's usually at least one decent choice.

8. Snack on fruits, vegetables, plain popcorn, pretzels, rice cakes and whole grain crackers. Not only are high-fat foods so dense in calories that you can blow your whole food plan with one handful of peanuts, but there is evidence that they affect the levels of serotonin in the body in a mood-altering way, often leading to depression and lethargy. Chocolate is the number one culprit.

Step Three: Increase Fiber

Fiber aids elimination and cuts the risk of colon and rectal cancers. It's also important in weight control, since fiber moves food more quickly through the digestive tract. High-fiber foods tend to be nutritional bonanzas.

These foods include whole grain breads and cereals, bran, fruits, vegetables, and beans, especially lima, navy, and kidney beans. But because these bottom-of-the-pyramid foods are so underrepresented in our diets, the average woman gets only 11 grams of fiber a day. She needs 20 to 30 grams for optimal health.

Begin with fruits and vegetables. To maintain maximum fiber, eat them raw or, if you prefer some vegetables cooked, either steam or microwave them. After a couple of weeks, move on to high-fiber breads or cereals. Bread should have two to three grams of fiber per serving, and if you don't like the taste of whole grains, there are fiber-enriched white and rye breads on the market. Cereal manufacturers have jumped on the fiber bandwagon with both feet, so you have a huge selection there. Look for five grams per serving, but remember that the one-ounce serving size listed on most cereal boxes is very small. If you're eating a whole bowl of cereal every morning, you're getting at least two servings; a fiber count of three grams per serving means you're actually eating closer to six.

Now for the beans. When planning one vegetarian meal per week, beans are a good place to start. Besides being high in fiber, they're low in fat and can form the base of many good soups, chilies, and Southwestern dishes.

Two words of warning: Don't introduce fiber all at once. If you go from 10 grams to 30 overnight, you may get sick. Start with the foods that are easier to digest, such as fruits and whole grain breads, and add the beans last. Also, fiber creates bulk, and unless that bulk is softened, you'll become constipated. Drink at least eight to ten cups of water a day.

7

❧

Wellness, Part Two: Detoxifying the Body, Stress Relief, and Natural Remedies

Detoxifying the Body

Eliminating Alcohol

There's no question that heavy drinking is bad for you, increasing your vulnerability to cancer, heart disease, liver disease, diabetes, and, of course, alcoholism. For women, drinking also brings a less publicized danger: alcohol interferes with your body's ability to absorb calcium.

Since heavy alcohol use often causes premature menopause, stopping estrogen production an average of five years earlier than normal, there's a doubled risk for women who drink. The earlier your menopause, the more years estrogen depletion weakens your bones. If alcohol also compromises your body's absorption of calcium, you have twice the average risk for osteoporosis.

Moderate drinking, which is usually defined as one or two drinks a day, isn't as dangerous. But some women report a glass of wine can trigger a hot flash. Moreover, two glasses of wine contain 200 to 250 calories, a sizable percentage of the 1,800 calories recommended daily for the average woman, and alcohol is nutritionally empty. An occasional 200-calorie splurge is not enough to blow your caloric total, but alcohol also lowers inhibition, resulting in the sort of what-the-hell attitude that can cause even the most fat-conscious woman to polish off a whole tray of nachos.

Some studies have indicated that even moderate drinkers show a heightened risk of breast cancer, although the percentage of increased risk is low. Drinking can also influence your sleep cycle; some women report that a glass of wine helps them get to sleep, but they then awake five hours later. For women who suffer from insomnia or disrupted sleep, alcohol only makes the goal of a good night's rest more elusive.

But even taking all this into consideration, there is some evidence that one drink a day might be good for you. A well-publicized study several years ago showed that, despite their high-fat diet and sedentary lifestyle, the French have a lower rate of heart disease than Americans. The theory is that red wine, which the French drink in abundance, increases the levels of good cholesterol, or HDL, in the blood. In the final analysis, a glass of wine when you're out for dinner is a relatively harmless indulgence, and it's only when you're having more than two drinks a day on a regular basis that your health begins to be compromised.

Eliminating Caffeine

In excessive amounts, caffeine can accentuate urinary stress incontinence, retard calcium absorption, and interfere with your ability to relax. (An excessive amount is defined as three cups of coffee or three soft drinks a day.) If you're prone to insomnia or irritability, switch to decaffeinated coffee and soft drinks.

Coming off caffeine can leave you dragging, especially if you're hooked on that morning cup of coffee. Make the change slowly by having caffeinated coffee for your morning drink and decaf for the rest of the day or by mixing the two for a low-caffeine blend for the first few weeks. There are some low-caffeine coffees on the market that can also help you bridge the gap.

Eliminating Nicotine

No need to equivocate here: Every study has shown that smoking is dangerous. Obviously, smoking sharply heightens your risk of lung cancer, and despite all the press about breast cancer, lung cancer remains the number one cancer killer of American women. Smoking, in fact, ultimately claims the life of 35 percent of the people who take up the habit, either through cancer or coronary disease. Would you fly an airline whose planes crashed one-third of the time? Considering how cautious we are in some areas of health care, our continuing tolerance of smoking is a case of a culture being in collective denial.

Nicotine works much like alcohol in the body, bringing on an earlier menopause and limiting calcium absorption. If a woman both smokes and drinks, she's likely to enter menopause prematurely, putting both her bones and her heart at risk far earlier than necessary.

Most smokers are well aware of the facts and have tried to quit, but nicotine is highly addictive, more so than many of the hard drugs we were warned about in college. Many women claim nicotine calms them, but as the effect of one cigarette wears off, they have to light another immediately or suffer the withdrawal jitters. Part of a smoking addiction is the amount of ritual involved; when the phone rings or after the last bite of a meal, smokers have subconsciously programmed themselves to reach for the pack.

The subconscious, however, can always be reprogrammed, and women often find help in support groups or through hypnosis or biofeedback. Those who find the physical aspects of the addiction more overpowering than the psychological might try weaning themselves off nicotine with skin patches or gum. Exercise is also an ally. People who begin an exercise program while giving up smoking are less likely to return to the habit than those who remain inactive.

For more information on quitting smoking, contact the American Cancer Society or the American Lung Association. Both are listed in the Sources section in the back of the book.

Stress Relief

The degree to which stress impacts our lives varies from woman to woman. We may all need the same amount of vitamins A and E, but how much R and R each woman needs depends on her lifestyle.

If you'll refer to the list of perimenopausal symptoms outlined in chapter 3, you can't help but notice how many of them are either caused or worsened by stress. You may live the life of an Olympian, but if you continue to worry, you're upping your chances of getting everything from colds to cancer. Even if you've never felt the need to learn stress reduction techniques before, perimenopause is definitely the time to expand your horizons.

Several of the women we surveyed mentioned that the stress of hormonal changes was intensified by life events (see Figures 7.1a and 7.1b). Change is inherently stressful so even a happy event such as marriage or a job promotion can take a toll on your nerves.

Just as many factors can cause stress, a variety of methods can alleviate it. Not everything on the following list will be your cup of tea, but keep an open mind, and eventually you'll find a stress-management technique that works for you.

Techniques for Managing Stress

Meditation   Classes in meditation and self-hypnosis will help you learn the basics, while various audiocassettes can lead you through progressive relaxation exercises. If you're feeling tense as well as suffering from memory lapses, try one of the energizing routines that are designed to leave you fresh and focused. If insomnia is a problem, using a relaxation tape to ease you into sleep is far preferable to relying on pills or alcohol to make you drowsy.

Self-hypnosis not only helps people relax and control anxiety but also counteracts some of the physical symptoms of perimenopause, including hot flashes. Since stress can trigger so many of the symptoms of perimenopause, self-hypnosis can intervene, breaking the maddening cycle of stress leading to a symptom, then the symptom leading to heightened stress.

Biofeedback   If your stress level is so high that it is causing anxiety attacks or physical illnesses such as migraines or ulcers, you need more help than conventional meditation offers. Biofeedback teaches you to use visualization and relaxation techniques to relieve physical problems and has proven exceedingly helpful in stress reduction.

For more information on biofeedback, contact the Biofeedback Society of America, listed in the back of the book.

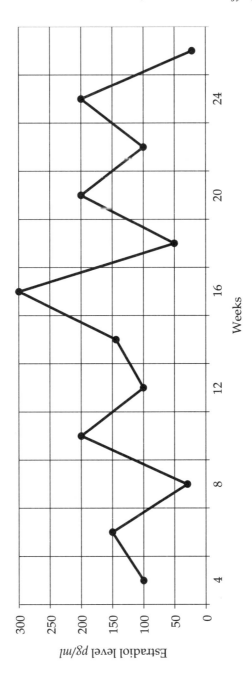

Figure 7.1a Variation in estradiol levels in the perimenopause.

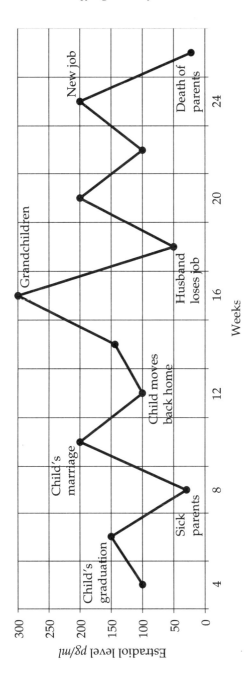

Figure 7.1b Life events of the perimenopausal woman.

Aerobic Exercise   It isn't necessary to exercise past the point of exhaustion or feel the celebrated "runner's high" to reap psychological benefits from exercise. Studies have shown that any regular aerobic activity releases endorphins that enhance your sense of well-being. People who exercise are also more apt to describe themselves as being in control and to feel a sense of mastery in all areas of their lives.

Yoga and T'ai Chi   Yoga is a system of physical exercises and stretches combined with deep breathing and relaxation. Many women turn to yoga as they age for the flexibility benefits, but it's an undeniable stress-buster as well. After years of being eclipsed by aerobics, yoga is making its way back into the mainstream. Your local exercise club or community college most likely offers a course, and even Jane Fonda has a yoga videotape out now.

T'ai chi, an exercise and breathing discipline that originated in China, is gaining popularity. Like yoga, there is an emphasis on breathing, body alignment, and flexibility, but t'ai chi is designed to stimulate as well as relax, making it an excellent wake-up routine. The exercise of choice for the elderly in the Orient, many people claim that t'ai chi is one reason that the Chinese enjoy enviably good health as they age, with much lower rates of cancer and arthritis than Americans in the same age group.

Even if you don't have time for a full-scale "Salute to the Sun" routine every morning, some of the techniques of these ancient traditions can easily be incorporated into a modern lifestyle. A few deep abdominal breaths during the day—at your desk, at a stoplight, while on the phone—can relieve tension and refresh you.

Massage   Nothing is more pleasurable than a good massage, and women who schedule massages on a regular basis report that they rest better and that their bodies release toxins more effectively, resulting in more regular elimination and clearer, younger-looking skin. As with the other relaxation techniques mentioned previously, it's worth going the professional route a few times to make sure you understand this treatment. Health spas and beauty salons often have a massage therapist on staff. After you get a sense of what a good massage is all about—no jerking, pinching, or excessive pressure—you may want to buy one of the videotapes or books on massage, invite a friend over and try it yourself. Aside from a relaxation technique, this can be an affectionate way to communicate with a friend or romantic partner.

Saunas, Hot Tubs, Whirlpool Baths   Relaxing after a workout is an important step in achieving the maximum benefits of exercise. Many health clubs have saunas and hot tubs, while growing numbers of people are opting to install whirlpools or hot tubs into their own homes. If you like the idea of massage but can't see spending time and money on regular appointments with a pro or if you lack a suitable massage partner, 20 minutes in your whirlpool tub can be a simple way of winding down before you go to bed.

Therapy and Support Groups   Menopause doesn't occur in a vacuum, and it is important to try to separate the hormonally induced problems from the life problems. Menopause can hit in the midst of divorce, financial setbacks, retirement or work dislocation, children leaving home, and all the other flotsam and jetsam of life.

Many women benefit from transition therapy during this hectic stage of their lives, and others find tremendous solace in joining a group of women who are going through similar disruptions. Debbie, a young cancer patient who appears in the final chapter of this book, credits the women in her postcancer support group with "saving her emotional life" and helping her to sort out which problems were due to her illness, which were due to chemotherapy, which to her premature menopause, and which were just general life junk. "I had reached the point where I'd lost all perspective," she says "and felt I was the only one who was going through this. My support group did more than any other single thing to bring my stress level down and teach me how to laugh again."

Speaking of laughter, you can employ a little self-therapy by taking in a funny movie, scheduling a weekend away, or just meeting a friend for lunch. Much of our tension is due to overwork, isolation from friends, and the frantic pace of our lives. Making a weekly date with yourself to hang out in a theater, museum, mall, or bookstore can go a long way toward reducing the treadmill feeling so familiar to women in mid life.

Menopause is the time to take care of *you*. It's important to learn to say no to demands on your time and to set aside an occasional afternoon or evening for yourself. This may mean resetting your priorities or standards about housekeeping, community service, and volunteering or reducing the time you spend in social activities you really don't enjoy. Recognize that you can't do it all and expect to live to be 80.

Even if you choose to handle your stress through the "head" method of group or individual therapy, don't forget that the mind-body connection is profound. You'll still benefit from exercise, relaxation tapes, massage, and the other stress-relievers we've discussed. The women who combat stress most effectively are those who take a multi-level approach.

Natural Remedies for Perimenopausal Symptoms

Women choose alternative or natural remedies to treat perimenopausal symptoms for several reasons. Their doctors may be patronizing or unresponsive to their needs. Symptoms in perimenopause tend to come and go in unpredictable patterns, and several women told us that each time they had made a doctor's appointment the troublesome symptoms would mysteriously abate a few days beforehand. Furthermore, rubbing yam cream on the abdomen is a simpler, less invasive treatment than full-throttle HRT and may seem more appropriate for a symptom that only appears for a few days each month. Some women cite philosophical reasons for taking the alternative path, such as their desire for greater control over their health care or their determination not to fool with Mother Nature.

The natural remedies listed here range widely in their effectiveness, depending upon the skill of the practitioner, the commitment of the user, and the general validity of the method.

As with any form of medicine, there are drawbacks to holistic treatments. Dosages are relatively uncontrolled, and the treatment regimes are based more on anecdotal evidence than scientific studies. That's not to say that what helped your neighbor's aunt won't help you, only that the outcomes of these treatments are less predictable than those of prescribed pharmaceuticals. Finally, these remedies are aimed at relieving specific symptoms and offer little help against potential bone and heart disease.

Homeopathy   Homeopathy is based on the belief that if some element in the body is out of balance, the best treatment is to supply more of the element that is causing this imbalance. For example, if you're troubled with nausea or gastrointestinal problems, a homeopathic physician might suggest small doses of ipecac. Ipecac, as you may remember if you ever child-proofed your home, induces vomiting if taken in large amounts.

At first the remedy may seem to make things worse, which, according to the homeopathic process, is proof that it's the right remedy. As balance is restored within the body and the symptoms gradually disappear, the remedy is taken in smaller and smaller doses and finally dropped altogether.

Homeopathy is a "whole body" approach. It often involves changes in diet, giving up toxins such as caffeine, nicotine, and alcohol, as well as the use of herbs.

Acupuncture   Calming, and nearly painless, acupuncture involves the placement of very thin needles into various parts of the body in order to stimulate the system. Acupuncture has proven helpful with stress, insomnia, and menstrual irregularity.

Needless to say, this is not a do-it-yourself methodology. Find a certified practitioner.

Primrose Oil   Despite the pleasant-sounding name, the oil used to relieve symptoms actually comes from salmon, tuna, and seeds. A brand that comes in capsule form is Efamol. Some women find primrose oil effective in treating bloating and cramps, as well as vaginal dryness.

Ginseng   The Korean ginseng root has been around through the ages. The Koreans and Japanese have taken this herb for centuries to procure energy and youthful vitality. In a dosage of 1,000 mg daily, many women claim it also helps hot flashes and night sweats. But don't overdo it. Ginseng is a stimulant, and ingesting too much can cause insomnia and anxiety.

Natural Progesterone   Wild Mexican yams contain a substance similar to progesterone, which relieves hot flashes. The yams come in pill, suppository, and cream form, but if you opt for the cream, be especially cautious about using it too frequently. Controlling dosages of a skin cream is nearly impossible, and excessive natural progesterone, like its synthetic counterpart, can lead to fluid retention, irritability, and weight gain.

B-6   This vitamin has long been recognized as a natural diuretic, helpful in reducing PMS-like symptoms, such as bloating and breast tenderness, and the attendant stress.

Vitamin E   In addition to being a valuable antioxidant, some devotees believe that vitamin E helps to relieve hot flashes. (Studies have yet to confirm the hot-flash claim.) The difference between using E as a vitamin supplement and using it as a natural remedy lies in the dosage. Naturalists advise 600 to 1,200 international units daily— far more than the 100 units recommended by the FDA or even the 400 recommended by the Alliance on Aging. Megadoses of vitamin E can lead to muscle weakness and fatigue, so don't exceed 1,000 units a day.

If you opt to take 400 units or more, add the mineral selenium, which facilitates the absorption of vitamin E. Otherwise most of the vitamin E will be lost in your urine.

Those with a strong interest in herbs and vitamins may want to read *The Change* by Germaine Greer. Ms. Greer lives in Europe, where natural remedies are more accepted and more widely used, and she offers detailed accounts of her own experiences with various herbs and homeopathic methods. *The Menopause Self Help Book* by Dr. Susan Lark also stresses a nonhormonal approach to menopause.

A Symptom-by-Symptom Guide to Natural Remedies

Hot Flashes
1. Try to isolate your "trigger foods," such as coffee, sugar, alcohol, or spicy foods, and then avoid them.
2. Exercise aerobically on a regular basis.
3. Helpful vitamin supplements include vitamin E, vitamin C, calcium, and selenium.
4. Herbs used in treatment include ginseng, sarsaparilla, dong quai, wild yam root, licorice root,

dandelion leaves, and alfalfa. Caution: Many of these herbs can be toxic in high dosages. Check with a homeopathic physician before you use them.

Vaginal Dryness

1. Use over-the-counter lubricants such as Astroglide, Gyne-Moistrin, Replens, Moist Again, Lubrin, or Today.
2. Remember the use-it-or-lose-it rule. Regular sex and/or masturbation increase the blood supply to the vagina, helping to prevent atrophy.

Insomnia or Night Sweats

1. Practice good sleep hygiene. Go to bed the same time every night. Avoid insomnia-producing foods and beverages like coffee, chocolate, and spicy dishes.
2. Get regular exercise—but not just before bedtime.
3. Use a soothing ritual—a hot bath, a massage, a few yoga postures, a progressive relaxation tape—to get you in the mood for sleep.
4. Avoid cigarettes and alcohol. They can disrupt your sleep cycle.
5. Helpful vitamin and mineral supplements include vitamins B, C, and E, zinc, copper, iodine, magnesium, and calcium.

Osteoporosis

1. Do weight-bearing exercises on a regular basis.
2. Take calcium supplements in the form of calcium carbonate or calcium phosphate.
3. Eat calcium-rich foods, which include milk, yogurt, cheese, and leafy, green vegetables.

4. Have a baseline DEXA when you are still in your 40s, then have regular follow-ups to make sure you're maintaining bone density.

Heart Disease

1. Eat a diet that is high in nutrients and fiber and low in fat. Have your cholesterol checked on a regular basis.

2. Exercise aerobically at least three times a week for a minimum of 30 minutes each time.

3. Maintain your ideal weight.

4. Don't smoke.

5. Drink only in moderation.

Attitude

The single most important component in wellness is attitude. When you see the impact of the changes you're making, the domino effect will begin to work for good instead of ill. In chapter 3, we discussed how one problem can lead to another, but it's equally true that one positive change can lead to another. Exercise makes you less likely to smoke. Giving up smoking makes it easier to exercise. In making dietary changes, you'll not only lose weight but your body will absorb more calcium and build bone and muscle mass, which in turn revs your metabolism and helps you keep the weight off. Utilizing relaxation techniques helps you to get a good night's sleep so you won't need your morning shot of caffeine. Because of the positive domino effect, you'll find that once you take the first step, all subsequent ones will be easier, resulting in a spiraling pattern of wellness.

8

Finding the
Right Doctor

Women are more likely to get their information on menopause from the news media or from friends than from a physician. We enter menopause much as we entered adolescence, with more "street knowledge" than hard facts.

Why don't women talk to their doctors? Sometimes it's just a lack of access. Many women approaching perimenopause may not have seen their gynecologist or family doctor for several years, particularly if they have finished bearing children and have permanent contraception. Perimenopause sneaks up on them, and they often try valiantly to ignore the symptoms. Even if they visit their doctor, the emphasis is on business as usual—Pap smears and breast checks—and they will downplay any symptoms or menstrual irregularity.

Since we're trained to deny menopause for as long as we can, the symptoms are probably pretty intrusive by the time a woman mentions them. That's one reason so many women are frustrated when they finally admit that "something's not right" but don't get much of a response from their doctor. Many gynecologists still buy into the definition of menopause as the cessation of menstruation and fail to connect the symptoms of a still-bleeding woman to hormone deprivation.

Even if you're one of the lucky few whose doctor recognizes the condition and uses the term *perimenopause,* your discussions are still likely to focus on your short-term symptoms. What you may get is a two-minute talk on hot flashes with little information on long-term health implications—and even less mention of mid-life sexuality or the emotional side effects of entering menopause.

In the final chapter, we'll hear several women's individual stories about the passage into perimenopause. Although their concerns and opinions vary widely, one striking commonality emerges from almost all of the stories: how awful their doctors were. The medical community's insensitivity toward menopausal women came up over and over again in the support groups we visited and among the women we interviewed. You can't assume your longtime physician will be up on the latest menopause theories or will even take your complaints seriously, but your chances for a successful dialogue improve if you approach the subject in the right way.

Schedule a Consultation

When you're climbing down from the stirrups after your annual Pap smear is hardly the best time to begin a discussion on perimenopause. Your doctor has 20 minutes blocked out for your appointment, so he or she may behave as if there's no time for your questions, simply because there isn't. It's not fair to either your doctor or yourself to try to squeeze a heavy discussion into the last minutes of a routine physical. This is not an "oh, by the way" issue.

A far better strategy is to schedule an appointment for a consultation concerning your perimenopausal symptoms. By asking the doctor to set aside time, you allow him or her to focus on the problem and you send a clear signal that you consider this important. Don't expect your physician to take your complaints seriously if *you* treat them as peripheral.

A consultation also goes a long way toward reducing the inequality inherent in most doctor-patient discussions. It's hard to feel you're being treated as a peer when you're lying naked on a table, speaking to someone above you who is fully dressed and clearly in a hurry. But if you meet over your doctor's desk, both sitting up, clothed, and with enough time to talk through the subject in detail, it's easier to establish the feeling of a partnership.

Your doctor should be able to explain how hormone replacement therapy is different for women in perimenopause than for those in menopause, help you to tally your individual risks for diseases or side effects, and discuss the pluses and minuses of various treatments. Your doctor should neither cheerlead for estrogen nor automatically reject it. During the consultation, you'll likely get a good sense of the depth of his or her interest in and knowledge of perimenopause, HRT, and the alternative treatments, and, just as importantly, you'll discover how comfortable you feel with him or her.

Prepare to pay as much or more for this session as for an annual physical. The consultation will take longer and involves a greater complexity of medical expertise and decision-making, both important factors in coding a visit for billing and insurance claims.

Is This the Right Doctor for You?

What's with all this "he or she" business? Does your doctor's gender matter? Many of the women with whom we spoke said they looked specifically for female doctors, because they found women physicians more empathetic. The more long-term and complex these women's treatments—in other words, the more visits they had to schedule—they more apt they were to insist that a woman physician be their guide.

Amanda, a woman we'll meet in the final chapter, was an active professional when she entered perimenopause. She not only traveled widely in her job but also held a rather high-profile position that required public speaking. She went to see her doctor when her periods had become so heavy that she was bleeding every day of the month. His response was a shrug and "I realize this might be an inconvenience. . . ." Amanda snorts at the memory. "Inconvenience! No woman professional would have dismissed another's problems with a comment like that." She ultimately found a female physician who appreciated the degree to which her symptoms were affecting her work, and, although it took several changes of medication, her periods are now regular.

This to not to imply that all male physicians are clods and all female physicians saints, only that, everything else being equal, you might feel more comfortable with a woman. Nonetheless, from this point on we'll refer to the physician as "he," not because we're sexist, but to make it semantically easier for readers to distinguish the doctor from the patient.

Issues of gender aside, how do you know whether your doctor is the right person to take you through perimenopause and beyond? If he won't agree to a consultation or seems to find this a bizarre request, that's your first clue something's wrong. Also, if his waiting room is exclusively populated by pregnant women, that should tip you off that he emphasizes the obstetric side of his practice and that non-pregnant and non-surgical patients won't get the same degree of attention.

During the course of your evaluation and treatment, some physicians will make statements that will send up red flags to tell you they don't have the right degree of expertise or interest. The following comments were actually made to women we surveyed; if you hear remarks like these, climb down from that table and head for the nearest exit.

Top 10 List of Physician Comments

10. "You're too young to be going through menopause."
9. "My wife takes these hormones and is doing just fine."
8. "Ask your friends what they use and let me know."
7. "Take this bag of hormone samples and see which one you like best."
6. "All women your age go through this. It's just something you have to put up with."
5. "The only problem is you're under too much stress."
4. "I don't start women on HRT until they haven't had a period for a year."
3. "I always . . ."
2. "I never . . ."
1. "I give up!"

What to Expect during an Office Visit

On your first visit, you can save your doctor a lot of time, and consequently save yourself a lot of money, if you bring a calendar or diary charting any menstrual irregularities you have experienced. Note such symptoms as hot flashes, sleep disturbances, mood swings, and headaches, as well as where they occur in your cycle. On a separate sheet of paper, list other symptoms that may not be tied to hormonal fluctuations, such as joint aches, vaginal dryness, irritability, and memory lapses.

Also be aware of the "misery index." How have these changes affected your quality of life? Do you miss days at work because of extremely heavy periods? Are you less effective on the job because of mood swings or nervousness? Is your relationship with your family changing? Has your sex drive diminished? If your misery index is low, just talking with your doctor and recognizing the stage of life you're entering may be adequate. However, if your work, relationships, or general self-esteem has begun to suffer, you need to discuss treatment alternatives.

The key word is *alternatives.* Be wary if your doctor claims he "always" treats his patients one way and it's "always" effective. If your doctor either tries to ram HRT down your throat or makes a blanket statement against it, recognize that he's more interested in selling a philosophy than in treating you as an individual.

Most doctors have a standard or pet regimen they try first, which is fine, but beyond that they should be flexible. The only thing worse than having a physician who pooh-poohs your symptoms is having one who uses a prefab treatment for every patient. The cartoon of the woman whose mouth has been taped shut with an Estraderm patch clearly illustrates that some doctors use HRT to silence a patient they perceive as just complaining. A physician truly committed to treating women at mid-life won't simply throw HRT at his patients; he'll help each one make the evaluation in the light of her entire health history. He should also be well-versed in how to combat symptoms via nutrition, exercise, and stress reduction. If a treatment doesn't work, the right doctor is willing to change the medication or the treatment; he won't argue that something must be wrong with the patient.

A tuned-in doctor will use this time to begin screening a woman for high cholesterol and breast cancer, if she isn't already having this done. Bone density tests should be considered for women at particular risk for osteoporosis. Contraceptive needs should be reevaluated. General health concerns regarding diet, nutrition, exercise, and smoking should be reassesed. Sometimes there are doubts about whether a woman is actually in menopause or not; FSH and estradiol tests may be helpful in making that determination.

If You Opt for HRT

Once a program of hormone replacement therapy is prescribed, the doctor or nurse should instruct you on how and when to take the pills, apply the patch, and so on. Calendars on which to mark break-through bleeding and other symptoms are helpful. You definitely should not be handed a prescription and told, "Good luck. Come back in a year." A follow-up visit in two to four months is necessary to evaluate your initial response to therapy, check for side effects, and review your bleeding pattern.

The third visit will be anywhere from six to nine months after beginning HRT, depending upon your response. Fine-tuning or even a complete change of medication is not uncommon in the first year of treatment and may be necessary again as you move through full-blown menopause.

Some practices have a nurse assigned to menopausal patients to answer their questions over the phone, deciding when they need to see the doctor versus needing minor changes in their medication versus needing simple reassurance.

Try not to confuse a cautious response with a lack of concern. Sometimes it's appropriate for the doctor to hold off on HRT to see whether the patient's misery index becomes high enough to warrant therapy. The physician must also separate the patient who is clinically depressed from the patient with perimenopausal mood swings. This is another good reason for an early follow-up visit; if the woman's mood has not improved on HRT, she may need to be referred for treatment for depression.

When Is It Necessary to See a Specialist?

Ideally, if your gynecologist, internist, or family doctor is having difficulty managing your symptoms, he'll refer you to a specialist before you become so frustrated that you decide to take your business elsewhere. You'll probably need a reproductive endocrinologist if:

♦ You're dissatisfied with the response you're getting from your doctor.

♦ You're in perimenopause and trying to conceive.

♦ Your symptoms are unusually pronounced or aren't responding to conventional treatment.

♦ You've had breast cancer or have an immediate-family history of the disease and need someone versed in the latest on HRT.

Many women find their specialists through word of mouth, and you're especially likely to be satisfied with your choice if you learn about him from another woman. Sharing information about doctors is one of the key benefits of a menopause support group. For a list of reproductive endocrinologists in your area, contact the American Fertility Society, listed in the Sources section of this book.

Seeing a specialist may require traveling to a medical center in another city. Women in suburban and rural areas don't always have easy access to specialists. The cost also can be prohibitive. But if you have a good relationship with your gynecologist or family physician, there is no reason to transfer all of your medical care to the specialist; many are available for diagnostic and planning consultations only. Most reproductive endocrinologists don't aim to provide ongoing gynecologic care but to get you settled on the proper regimen and then refer you back to your regular physician.

The term "specialist in menopause" is not a synonym for "specialist in hormone replacement therapy." A menopause specialist should be able to tailor a plan of management for the woman who doesn't want to take hormones, focusing on increased calcium, vitamin therapy, a lowfat diet, and exercise, with monitoring for heart disease, osteoporosis, and breast cancer.

9

Psychology, Sexuality, and Perimenopause

Let's forget for a moment about how perimenopause affects your body and focus on how it affects your mind. Even the women we surveyed who claimed to know nothing about menopause didn't hesitate to venture theories in this area—that menopause is a factor in mental illness, that it instantly makes a woman less sexual, that it is the first step in the descent into old age.

It's undeniable that hormones have an impact on both mood and sexuality, as any woman who has gone into sudden estrogen deprivation can attest. But we are more than our hormones, and it is equally undeniable that our moods are influenced by many factors, not the least of which is our expectations. Menopause is often a self-fulfilling prophecy: a woman who believes it marks the end of youth will be more apt to blame every marital spat and memory lapse on menopause than a woman who has a more positive mind-set. In this chapter, we'll try to separate the problems that can accurately be attributed to menopause from those that cannot, and offer suggestions on how to deal with both.

Several of the women with whom we spoke mentioned that they weren't aware of how much their personalities had changed during perimenopause until either someone else pointed it out or they looked at themselves in retrospect. "My kids kept telling me I was edgy," they said, or "I see now it was probably perimenopause that was making me so antisocial." During the time in which the changes are happening, it can be tough to be objective about your own condition.

Does Perimenopause Cause Depression?

Menopause, contrary to myth, doesn't cause depression.

We muddy the water in these discussions with our tendency to use the term *depression,* which is a specific and serious illness, as if it meant "in a bad mood" or "a little down." Estrogen deprivation can trigger a bad mood or sap your energy, but it does not bring on full-scale clinical depression.

Clinical depression is twice as common in women as in men, which is possibly the root of the misconception that menopause and mental illness are synonymous terms. But separate studies in the United States, England, and Sweden have all shown that women are no more prone to have their first bout of depression during menopause than at any other time. *Involutional melancholia,* once a catchall phrase that implied any mental problems found in women over the age of 40 were hormonal, has been removed as a diagnostic classification in the psychiatric manual.

This is not to say that estrogen, or a lack of it, doesn't affect your mood. When estrogen levels fall from their high during pregnancy, for example, 50 to 70 percent of women experience a mild, transient depression over the first 10 days after delivery, 10 to 20 percent develop a significant postpartum depression, and a tiny number—less than one-tenth of one percent—develop major psychosis.

Likewise, when estrogen levels drop during perimenopause, many women experience mood swings and 65 percent of the women attending menopause clinics report feelings of mild depression. Often these moods are related to another symptom; if a woman's hot flashes and night sweats are so disruptive that she hasn't had a good night's sleep in a month, it's no surprise that she finds herself teary and on edge.

Hormonal depression usually involves feelings of lethargy, a lack of concentration, less interest in sex, and perhaps less desire to socialize. HRT helps the vast majority of the women troubled with hormonal depression, both because it relieves the underlying symptoms and because estrogen has a mood-altering effect on the brain. Specific receptors for estrogen are located in the limbic forebrain, the area that is responsible for our emotions. Estrogen increases the levels of serotonin, a chemical associated with good moods. In fact, by counteracting the chemicals that limit serotonin production, estrogen acts similarly to the antidepressant Prozac.

It's important to remember that we're talking about using HRT to treat relatively minor depression and mood swings, not true despair. A woman who goes into her doctor's office with thoughts of suicide or a complete inability to function is not suffering from hormonal depression and should not be immediately started on HRT. Estrogen can make the situation worse. Clinical depression is a life-threatening condition that requires psychiatric evaluation and therapy. HRT can be started, if needed, only after the illness is under control.

Are Mood Swings Worse When Menopause Is Abrupt?

Usually. Women who undergo an unusually rapid menopause, whether natural or medically induced, are at higher risk for depression than women who undergo menopause gradually. Their estrogen withdrawal is sudden, similar to what women experience after childbirth, leading to a hormonal crash. (Not to mention that recovery from major surgery or cancer is emotionally draining in itself.) Some women who have gone through an abrupt menopause also report that their sex drive decreases dramatically; they may benefit from the addition of small amounts of testosterone to their HRT regimen.

Is It All Hormonal?

As we've seen, many of life's stresses hit during perimenopause. A woman in her 40s may be experiencing kids moving out, kids moving back in, the responsibility of caring for aging parents, divorce, job loss or relocation, loss of friends, mixed feelings about getting older, and, as one woman put it, "a real resentment that my body suddenly seems to be turning on me."

Several of the women with whom we spoke specifically mentioned feeling out of control, as if their bodies had an agenda of their own. A 40-year-old woman in perimenopause may have a harder time with this control issue than a woman in her 50s, since the younger woman is dealing with a whole array of symptoms she didn't expect for another 10 years. Of course, no one wants a hot flash in the middle of a sales presentation, irregular periods while on a business trip, or to find themselves dealing with sub-fertility as the biological clock is ticking loudly.

An interesting statistic to ponder: richer women report more menopausal symptoms than poorer women, no matter what country they live in. It seems paradoxical. Why would women with good nutrition, more education, and better access to health care have the most problems?

At first glance, this fact would seem to lend credence to the theory that women are just bitching, that the more money a woman has, the more leisure time she has to obsess about her symptoms. But this statistic more likely means that when it comes to feeling good, poor people have lower expectations. Poor women will typically suffer much longer than middle-class women before they seek medical help and, in the presence of a doctor, often downplay the intensity of their symptoms. A hot flash may seem like a minor complaint relative to the sound of gun-fire outside the apartment window.

Perimenopausal moodiness may also be tied to a woman's expectations about aging. In cultures such as China's, where the elderly are honored, few menopausal symptoms are reported. This could be because of differences in the Chinese diet and lifestyle—or it could be because Chinese women are proud to grow older. In the U.S., lesbians are less troubled by menopausal symptoms than heterosexual women, and lesbian couples report no decline in libido or frequency of sexual activity.

We could speculate for days on why these differences exist, but in the meantime it's beyond question that menopause is doubly rough on women who live in a culture that is both male-dominated and youth-oriented. Our society—from the anxious articles on how to understand men that fill women's magazines to the sensationalized media reports on how few suitable unattached men there are—equates a woman's self-worth with her ability to attract and hold a man. If a woman is indifferent to male perceptions of her, menopause may be inconvenient, but it probably isn't scary. On the other hand, if a woman feels she is competing for male attention with younger, more "hormonally advantaged" women, her fears about aging may become strong enough to literally make her sick.

Plastic Surgery

Now you may be asking, "So, assuming I'm not a lesbian in Beijing, I should visit a plastic surgeon? Is that your point?"

We're describing, not prescribing. Assuming they can afford it, perimenopause is indeed a time when many women resort to plastic surgery. Common procedures include an abdominoplasty, or tummy tuck, which removes the loose skin from previous pregnancies, and breast reconstruction. Women may also opt to have a face-lift, skin peels, or collagen injections to plump out facial wrinkles.

A relatively new type of operation, liposuction, has become the most common plastic surgery procedure in the U.S. Liposuction is not a cure for general obesity—an average of four pounds is sucked out in a standard procedure—nor is it a substitute for diet and exercise. But since body fat distribution is largely hereditary, some otherwise slender women have pads of fat on their hips, thighs, or abdomens. Liposuction is used to remove the fat cells from these isolated places and improve the body contours.

Some women find the idea of plastic surgery offensive, the result of unrealistic and sexist cultural demands that 50-year-olds look like 30-year-olds. They matter-of-factly point out that men do not feel a corresponding pressure to hide their sags and bags, and assert that America has gone overboard in its worship of youth. Other women just as matter-of-factly point out that when they look better they feel better—so why not? One woman we interviewed, who has had four separate reconstructive procedures and is not yet 50, argued that the emphasis on the mind-body connection is usually given to how we can use our minds to improve our bodies. "But it works both ways," she says. "If you improve your body, it helps your mental attitude."

Since you'll bring your own value judgments to the issue, it remains, like so many of the topics we've discussed, a deeply private choice. Two things are certain: As we baby boomers move through middle age, plastic surgery is going to continue to be big business, and our society's attitude toward aging women is going to remain a hot topic.

Talking to Your Partner

Without getting into the overdone issue of the male midlife crisis, it's worth mentioning that if your partner is having his own troubles adjusting to aging, this will influence how well you cope. If your husband dreads the thought of getting old, you may even wonder whether you should try to hide your complaints from him.

Yet a woman in menopausal transition needs to be open with her partner about her symptoms and how they're affecting her emotions, energy level, and sexual interest. Just as many women wait to see their doctors until the symptoms have become unbearable, they often wait to broach the subject with their partners until they're at the emotional breaking point.

Men certainly have no intrinsic undertanding of menopause, so an explanation of just what a hot flash is may be called for, along with telling him what you're doing to address the problem. We've already discussed that women don't like feeling out of control. Not surprisingly, men hate it too. If your husband seems indifferent to your symptoms, it may be because he feels helpless and is wondering, "Why are you telling me this if I can't do anything about it?" An unemotional, results-oriented man will respond better to a conversation that basically says, "Here's what's going on with me . . . and here's what I'm doing to combat it."

In addition, it may help to express what's positive about the approaching time of life—no more need for birth control, no more periods or PMS. If you're instituting changes in your diet, starting to exercise, or learning stress-management techniques, invite him to participate. Then the focus moves from your menopause into the broader sphere of what you both can do to make the coming years as terrific as possible. Aging isn't just about the negatives; it's also about travel, leisure, new hobbies, and more time to enjoy each other.

Frequency of Sexual Activity

And now you may be muttering, "OK, OK. We'll take up golf, but our sex life is over, right?"

Different, maybe. But not over.

There is an age-related decline in the frequency of intercourse for both men and women, but menopausal women decrease their sexual activity more than men of the same age. In one study, 7 percent of women between the ages of 45 and 50 stated they have "no interest in sex." This increased to 20 percent for 51 to 55-year-olds and to 31 percent by ages 56 to 60. Although many authors (and many husbands) attribute this decline in interest among women to changes in male function and behavior, studies haven't borne this out. Sexual frequency seems to be more tied to the woman's interest level than the man's, with little connection to either the male's age or level of interest.

Just as most heart disease studies have focused on male subjects, so have most studies on mature sexuality, so the question of why these women lose interest in sex has never been fully addressed. Much has been made of the differences in male arousal time that come with age: it takes a man three seconds to get an erection at age 18, 18 to 20 seconds at age 45, and five minutes, or more, at age 75. But, let's face it, among all the complaints women have about men, "They're too slow sexually" doesn't usually make the top 10. How many women really care about this slowdown, unless they have a train to catch?

Men earnestly believe that women change in response to their changes—after all, our entire sexuality exists in response to theirs, right? But most women say that their lack of interest has more to do with what's going on inside them than with changes in their partners. Some women report that menopause does bring on a decline in desire while others confess that they're playing the myths about menopause to their own benefit, using them as an excuse to forgo sexual activity after what may have been years of indifference.

Studies show that rates of sexual activity fall steadily for both women and men from the ages of 20 to 40, but after 40, the decline becomes dramatic. One study reported a decrease from 59 "episodes" per year at age 38 to 26 per year by age 50. In other words, by her late 40s, a woman may be having sex less than half as often as she was at the beginning of her 40s. (It's important to remember that these statistics are based on some nonexistent "average" man and woman; some couples have sex rarely or never, while others, especially if their level of general marital satisfaction is high, have sex as often as they ever did.)

In this chapter, much as in the early chapter on fertility, we may seem to be making the false assumption that every perimenopausal woman is in a relationship. We realize that women may go through years without a suitable partner, or even an unsuitable one, and sometimes the frequency of sex declines through lack of opportunity. If you aren't currently in a sexual relationship, even if you have no plans to have one in the future, read on. Your vaginal health is still important, and most of the benefits of sexual stimulation, such as increased glandular and blood activity in the pelvic region, can be just as easily achieved through masturbation as intercourse. Stimulation and orgasm, not the mere presence of a partner, maintain vaginal tissue.

Physical Changes in the Genitals

When ovarian function ceases, the woman loses both estrogen and testosterone. The loss of testosterone can dampen sexual enthusiasm, although in some women the effect is more pronounced than in others. The loss of estrogen, however, actually affects physiology. The following descriptions are not designed to terrify you. Just as with any other symptom, some women report the condition to a much greater degree than others and some women are unaffected.

The first changes you're apt to notice are in the outer genitals. Pubic hair thins and the labia loses fat tissue, meaning your vaginal lips become less full and less responsive to touch. Inside, the walls of the vagina thin and become more fragile as a result of the decreased blood supply. If the vagina is not stimulated through sexual play or masturbation, the diminished circulation will eventually affect the nerves and glands.

As the nerves lose function, there is less sensation during intercourse, and as the glands lose function, there is less lubrication. Needless to say, many women at this point are avoiding intercourse, thinking, "Why bother?" But abstinance accelerates the cycle of deterioration. The phrase "use it or lose it" may sound unsympathetic, but it's accurate.

If the early warning signs go untreated, the vagina will become smaller and less elastic. This condition is known as vaginal atrophy. If a woman with vaginal atrophy attempts to have intercourse, she will find that, between the decreased lubrication and the decreased elasticity, her vagina does not lengthen to accommodate the man's penis as it used to do. At best, she feels nothing. At worst, she feels pain. In the very worst-case scenario, the walls of the vagina can tear during intercourse.

As if all this weren't enough, the acid-base balance of the vagina also changes, and new higher pH level makes it more susceptible to infections. An atrophied vagina is much more likely to become inflamed and to develop itching, discharge, and seemingly endless minor infections. Having vaginitis 40 weeks of the year can profoundly depress what's left of your sexual desire.

Even if the vagina does not deteriorate completely, once estrogen depletion has begun to alter a woman's physiology, response to sexual stimulation becomes muted. One woman reported that it felt as though she were having sex while fully dressed—like a layer of cloth was between her skin and her husband's. Besides the loss of skin receptivity, there is also less preorgasmic muscle tension and a delay in the reaction time of the clitoris, making a woman only half as likely to have an orgasm as she used to be.

Twenty-one percent of perimenopausal women report that they have an orgasm every time they have sex, but only 10 percent of postmenopausal women climax every time. Menopause is only part of the reason. As a woman ages, her general health may decline (as may her partner's), and she is more likely to be taking medications, such as antihypertensives or even antidepressants like Prozac, that inhibit sexual response.

After reading this laundry list of miseries, you may feel like taking a Prozac yourself, but take heart. Even if things are changing down below, the brain remains the chief sexual organ. Happily married and newly married women in mid-life report that they crave sex as much as they ever did, and the previously cited reports about lesbians and women who live in cultures that celebrate aging only serve to underscore that attitude is everything. If physiology were the sole component of sexuality, we would all lose interest in sex at the same time and at the same rate. Obviously, we don't.

While your attitude toward sex has little to do with whether or not you experience the physical changes just described, it has everything to do with what happens after any changes occur. Women who are essentially uninterested in sex will welcome an excuse to terminate their sex lives; women who want to have sex will find a way to overcome the physical barriers.

How to Combat these Changes

HRT increases vaginal lubrication and reverses the thinning of the vaginal walls, relieving painful intercourse. Since sex doesn't hurt anymore, desire in turn reawakens and sexual frequency returns to premenopausal levels.

If you're trying to avoid HRT, start with an over-the-counter lubricant, such as Replens or Astroglide. While it will not reverse thinning or damage to the vaginal walls, a lubricant without estrogen will make sex comfortable enough to enjoy, and, since sex increases the blood supply to the area, a lubricant can get the cycle turning once again in a more positive direction.

The key is not to wait too long before seeking intervention. Your doctor can test for vaginal dryness and atrophy, but by the time problems show up in a routine exam, they're pronounced. Only you know how much you naturally lubricate, how much you think or fantasize about sex, and how sex usually feels to you, so you will obviously

be the first one to notice any changes. If lack of lubrication or decreased vaginal sensation is your only symptom,
you may just require an estrogen cream to make sex fun
again. But don't convince yourself that it's all in your
head and that desire will return on its own in a month or
two. If you avoid sex or masturbation altogether, you'll
lose whatever elasticity and response you have left.

Will Your Sex Life Be the Same?

There's a variation on an old joke: When filling out a sur-
vey on menopause, a woman reports that she hasn't had
an orgasm since entering menopause. Her doctor is concerned and changes her medication, adds testosterone,
and advises the use of lubricants. After months without
improvement, she happens to mention that she never had
an orgasm before menopause either.

HRT can't correct a problem that existed prior to
menopause, and this may be a good time to rethink your
entire approach to sex. After all, the statistic mentioned
earlier—that only 21 percent of premenopausal women
regularly experience orgasm—illustrates that most
women aren't reaching their full pleasure potential even
before hormone withdrawal becomes an issue.

Many couples benefit from counseling during this
transitional phase, and innumerable books on the market
deal with the subject of mid-life sexuality. *Sex Over 40* by
Saul Rosenthal, M.D., provides information on the effects
of menopause and male hormonal changes, common
drugs that may affect sexuality, as well as intercourse positions for people who suffer from arthritis, osteoporosis, or
joint problems. Although it does not focus specifically on
any age group, *For Each Other: Sharing Sexual Intimacy* by
Lonnie Barbach, Ph.D., does an excellent job of address-
ing the issues of diminished desire and the powerful
effect the mind can have on sexuality.

We spoke with women who changed partners, changed attitudes, and even changed their sexual orientation during this time of their lives. While your transition might be less dramatic, it's important to keep an open mind. Many women with whom we spoke pointed out that if you are looking for a new partner in this stage of life, the old constraints may no longer apply. You're less likely to be looking for a man to father your children or to give you social acceptability or financial security. Your primary requirement in a mid-life relationship may just be "the pleasure of their company" a factor frequently mentioned by women who ended up with a younger man, another woman, or someone they would never have considered a likely partner in their youth.

Because the focus is on how the other person makes them feel, women in mid-life may make more adventurous choices than those they made 30 years earlier. If you do seek a new sexual partner, remember to be vigilant about birth control and to use a condom, either the male or female type, if there is the slightest chance of exposure to venereal disease.

Even if you're in a long-term relationship or marriage, medical conditions may force you to look for new ways to express your sexuality. The standard missionary position is not the best for a woman suffering from osteoporosis or vaginal atrophy; if she is on top she can control the depth of penetration and won't have to support her partner's weight. If your husband has back or joint problems of his own, rear entry or side-by-side positions can keep you from hurting him.

This may be the time to consider how many burdens you can remove from each other in every sense, a time to become more playful and experimental. If a male partner is bothered with impotence or less-than-firm erections, oral sex will work better than intercourse, since it relieves him from pressure to perform. Because the stimulation is more direct, oral sex also is a good alternative as a woman's sexual response time lengthens.

And, of course, the statistics don't reveal it all. Frequency is not the only component in sexual satisfaction, and some couples report that they're doing it less, but enjoying it more. Sexuality flourishes for many women in their 50s and 60s, especially when they're willing to be more creative. Menopause marks the end of your reproductive life, but the best years of your sexual life may still be ahead.

10

Talking with Other Women

Benefits of a Support Group

Do you need a support group to help you through peri-menopause? At first glance the question may seem ridiculous. You're busy. You have friends. Do you really want to drive across town to hang out with a group of women when all you have in common is menstrual irregularity?

A support group doesn't have to be a formal organization associated with a hospital or clinic; we spoke with one group that evolved out of a bunch of high school friends promising to stay in touch after their 25th reunion. If you would describe your perimenopausal experience as "typical," a support network of friends may be all you need. Women with more specialized problems, however, such as those experiencing premature menopause or severe symptoms, will probably benefit from joining a focused group. If you're having a difficult time in menopause, you need to be around other women whose experiences mirror yours, not well-meaning friends assuring you that it's all in your head.

Whether you opt to join an organized group or just be more open with your friends, don't underestimate the importance of female bonding. Women who have other women to whom they can talk do much better than those who attempt to go through this particular rite of passage in silence. One of the key consequences of a group is shared information—the name of a sympathetic doctor, a debate on the benefits of patches versus pills, techniques on fighting sleeplessness. Women collectively also can lobby for changes in the health-care system with more authority than we can muster as individuals.

Many hospitals and women's clinics offer support groups, which are often made up of women who share a specific medical condition such as premature menopause, cancer, or infertility. If your needs are more general, you might fit in with a group whose roots are a local women's organization, church, synagogue, or community center. A large city will have more than one group, with origins typically as diverse as the Junior League, a Catholic parish, and the local chapter of the National Organization for Women, making it easy to find one that fits your personal style.

Once you get through the door, you'll probably find you have more in common with the group members than hot flashes. Women who tackle menopause head-on tend to be dynamic, proactive, interesting people, who don't take aging lying down. "We consider ourselves hormonally challenged, not hormonally handicapped," one woman told us, laughing. Another group told a funny story about how an invited speaker asked them whether they had any questions and they looked at each other, shaking their heads. "We knew we'd meant to ask the next speaker about something," they said. "But when it came time for the questions, we all went blank." The next morning they remembered that what they had all forgotten to ask about was their memory loss.

One woman in the group confided that, when she was alone, her lapses in concentration were anything but amusing and that there were times when she felt almost panic-stricken, "like I was losing my mind." Being in the group reassured her that her symptoms were normal and helped her rediscover her sense of humor. The group made a big banner that read, "Remember that we've lost our memory," and hung it on the wall for the next meeting.

"So many of the questions," explains the woman with the memory problem, "revolve around a single concern: 'Is this normal?' Often we answer that question among ourselves before the expert even shows up. The answer is usually 'Yes, it's normal. I'm going through it too.'"

If you would like to start your own perimenopause support group, it can be as simple as finding a group of friends, taking turns meeting in each other's homes, and picking a discussion topic each month. For information on how to start a group or find an existing one, write or call the North American Menopause Society, listed in this book's Sources section, or contact a women's clinic or hospital in your area.

The Women's Stories

Every woman's transition into menopause is different, and nothing illustrates this more powerfully than the stories of the individual women we interviewed. We selected several women who went through the change in their own ways and asked them what they would like to say to other women about their experiences. Consider this a support group on paper.

Claudia

"Who was this person who was always crying, tired all the time? I was willing to do anything it took to get my old self back."

Claudia, an attractive, confident woman who used to be a fashion model, is the antithesis of the menopausal granny. She and her husband travel extensively for their import-export business and have two college-age sons, and Claudia has lived on four continents.

"We'd moved with the kids nine times in our marriage and I thought I could handle change," she says wryly. But she was unprepared when, at 50, her periods suddenly stopped. "Within four months I went from being completely regular to having no bleeding at all. I felt like I had PMS all the time. I was tired, bloated, crying over anything, and anxious about ridiculous things." Although Claudia's everyday life was stressful enough to stop most women in their tracks, she never once felt that her changes in attitude were connected to anything but her hormones.

"I enjoy a fast pace," she says, "assuming I can get a good night's rest. But once I went into menopause, I had night sweats so bad that I was waking up dripping wet and unable to go back to sleep. It went on night after night, and I haven't felt anything like that level of exhaustion since my boys were babies. Within six weeks, my nerves were so ragged I was unable to work. I've always been appearance-conscious, but suddenly I was fighting a losing battle. I was too bloated to wear half my clothes, my skin and hair were dry, and I had bags under my eyes."

Claudia's longtime doctor described her complaints as "typical" and advised her to "grin and bear it." A second doctor put her on an estrogen skin patch, which she has used for five years with great success. "Within six weeks on estrogen, the hot flashes stopped, I was resting better and had my energy back," she says. "I resent even those few months I felt so bad because it wasn't necessary.

"The thing is, my mother's life was predictable. She died in the same town she was born in. She expected to age at a certain rate, expected to die at a certain age, and, frankly, nothing much was required of her after menopause. She ended up living with two of her sisters. After lunch, they would go lie down and pull the shades.

"But my life is unpredictable. I work, I travel, my siblings and I all live in different countries. The society I'm in happens to be preoccupied with youth, which is regrettable in many ways, but in another way it is good for me. I couldn't go into a bedroom at noon and pull the shades even if I wanted to. There's too much I'm expected to do."

Annie

"As long as I can avoid doctors and drugs, I will. My past experiences have all been bad."

Annie, a 46-year-old teacher with a teenage daughter, has been in perimenopause for at least eight years. "My body's always been off the normal pace," she shrugs. "I started my periods at the age of nine and was skipping periods and having hot flashes by my late 30s. I still have them, but they're very irregular and very heavy and sometimes go on for a month at a time."

Although this menstrual roller coaster has drained her energy, Annie is reluctant to consider HRT. "I'm extremely phobic about drugs. They're not natural. I have a history of reactions, bad side effects. I won't even take an aspirin unless I'm absolutely desperate."

She has even more reservations about doctors than about drugs. "No one has ever talked to me," she says flatly. "It's just 'Do you want this pill or not?' No explanations, no options, just a prescription. My doctor will not

acknowledge my fears or even answer my questions."
Twice worn down by periods that lasted for weeks, she got
a prescription for estrogen but never had either filled. "I
kept thinking I'd give it another day or two, and both
times I stopped bleeding on my own.

"I can handle short-term symptoms like hot flashes,
even the marathon periods, if I have to. But there's a lot
of heart disease in my family and I do wonder sometimes
about the long-term effects. I'll be living a very long time
without estrogen. . . . It's not that I like wearing a pad
every day of my life. It seems like stubbornness, but it's
really more a lack of information. I won't take anything
until I have to, and I'll never take anything I don't understand. And so far I can't find anyone who can explain
estrogen to me."

Amanda

"I'm using a combination of traditional medical solutions,
like estrogen, along with alternative remedies like acupuncture and stress reduction. I pick and choose among
everything that's available."

"When I went to my gynecologist, I was 44, about to be
married and pretty sure I was going into menopause," says
Amanda. "It was not exactly the greatest time to be losing
interest in sex and having vaginal dryness. He looked at
my chart, not at me, and totally laughed off the idea of
menopause. I asked him about estrogen, and he said,
'You're too young.' He seemed insulted by my questions,
like the very fact I was interested in my health care meant
I was doubting his expertise or judgment."

"I told him about the vaginal dryness, and he said,
'You're depressed.' I said I was a therapist and I'd know if
I was depressed, thank you very much." She bristles at the
memory. "When I told him about my menstrual cramp-

ing, all he could say was that he'd do a D and C. Evidently that's his standard cure."

Wary of surgery and furious that her doctor didn't seem to trust her opinions about what was happening in her body, Amanda searched out a new gynecologist, a younger woman. "My new doctor is the first person I ever heard use the term perimenopause," she says. "We had a long interview during which time she asked a lot of questions about my medical history and laid out all the options. Finding the right physician is so important because, believe me, this is a long-term relationship. It took me four changes of medication before I found the combination that worked. If you don't have faith in your doctor, you'll never get through the process.

Although HRT relieved many of her symptoms, her experience with her first doctor demonstrated to Amanda the need to take full responsibility for her own medical care. As a therapist, she was well aware of the effect stress can have on physical problems, and she began seeking alternative remedies as well as conventional treatment. Acupuncture has helped with her menstrual cramps, and she uses a variety of self-relaxation techniques to cope with the demands of everyday life. "I don't have an agenda when it comes to medical care," she says. "I tell my M.D. about the acupuncture and my friends at the health food store about the estrogen. I'll use whatever works."

Lynn

"Menopause was a breeze."

"I'm not really sure when menopause happened," says Lynn, a 49-year-old writer with children aged 11 and 9. "I was on birth control pills, and at some point my hormones must have just gradually tapered off." Now off the Pill, Lynn remembers "a couple of hot flashes and some vaginal dryness, which she handled with an over-the-counter lubricant. She is not eager to take HRT. "I enjoy not having periods," she says.

Although she feels great and is able to juggle the demands of job and family with enviable ease, Lynn occasionally worries about aging. "There's lots of osteoporosis in my family," she says. "My mother had the hump. My sister is absolutely religious about taking calcium, and I keep meaning to buy a bottle.

"Some things about aging have been tough for me. Both of my parents are dead, and sometimes I come face to-face with my own mortality. But menopause was easy. I don't mourn the loss of my ability to bear children, and my sex life is better than ever. I think that if you don't have the physical symptoms, it's easy not to think about the emotional issues, and since I never had this big bang, this moment of 'Oh, I'm in menopause,' I don't really feel all that changed. It's OK to say that, isn't it? That for me menopause was no big deal?"

Debbie

"Over the past year, I've been diagnosed with cancer, had chemotherapy, and gone into menopause. I had to let go of the control issue. Things I never could have predicted were happening to my body, and all I could do was respond to them. Feeling powerless was the worse part."

Debbie was 33 when chemotherapy following lymphatic cancer destroyed her ovaries and threw her into an immediate menopause. "My ovaries were dead by the second chemo treatment," she says. "I had the whole package within two weeks—hot flashes, vaginal dryness, insomnia, depression."

Debbie's doctor nagged her until she overcame her lethargy and joined a hospital support group designed for women in chemotherapy-induced menopause. "After the meeting," she remembers, "for the first time in a long time I considered myself lucky. I have a child, but two of the women in the group had gotten cancer while they were in their 20s and single. On top of everything else, they had tremendous anger over the loss of their child-bearing potential."

Debbie's new friends helped her wade through the arduous process of trying to determine which symptoms were related to the cancer, which to the chemotherapy, which to the stress, and which to menopause. "I was tired, weepy, had absolutely no interest in sex and horrible memory loss, the kind where you'd start writing a check and literally forget your own name. At first I blamed everything on the chemo. But after the chemo was wrapped up and I was still having the symptoms, I had to say 'Wait a minute. . . .'"

The fact that so many of her symptoms seemed interconnected made it hard for Debbie to figure out what was causing what, much less how to tackle the problem. Was the depression hormonal—or because she'd had cancer? Was the depression killing her sex drive—or was it the leftover toxins from the chemo causing her vaginal dryness? "Having cancer is so overwhelming that you focus completely on it," she says. "I'm not sure I would have connected any of the symptoms to a loss of estrogen if it hadn't been for the other women. Collectively we were having so many of the same things happen to us that as time passed we kept sharing information and finding answers as a group."

Working closely with her doctor and bouncing ideas off her support group, Debbie has begun trying various combinations of HRT and natural remedies. "If you're in a premature menopause," she concludes, "you have to work to get over the control issue. If I hadn't been able to come to terms with the fact that things were happening to me beyond my control, I never would have been able to move on. My sense of isolation was heavy—not that many women in their 30s have to deal with what I'm dealing with—but my support group saved my life."

Peggy

"I found women reluctant to band together and accept the label *menopausal.*"

"I disappointed myself in how I reacted to aging," admits Peggy, an energetic 51 year old executive and new lywed. "I thought I was above being bothered by it, but I discovered in my 49th year that I was bothered big-time about it."

Peggy's epiphany came on a vacation with her daughter, when a man approached their table in a restaurant and asked if he could join them. "He was maybe 10 years younger than me, easily 20 years older than my daughter," Peggy recalls, "and it took me half the meal to realize it was her he was interested in, not me. I thought, 'This is it. The torch has passed on to the next generation. I'm invisible.'"

When Peggy first began experiencing menopausal symptoms at the age of 46, she attributed them to stress. "I called it a malaise," she says. "My job is so intense that I connected the insomnia and exhaustion to work. All of a sudden I didn't want to be around people, even though I'm people-oriented. I had no sexual energy." A pause. "That's not like me. My incontinence was so bad that I was wearing Depends, but the memory lapses were even more humiliating. I'd sit down with a monthly expense sheet at work and just go blank, have no idea why I'd picked it up or what I was looking for."

It was the hot flashes, however, that became so intense she could no longer explain them away and that ultimately drove her to her doctor. "He gave me a patch. No questions, no discussion. I'd been going to him for 14 years, and he still wasn't listening to me. He made his money delivering babies, and he didn't have time for my picky, pesky problems. I sat there on the table and thought, 'I'm going to dump this guy.'" Like Amanda, she found a woman doctor more empathetic, but it still took two years to get the medication right. "Lots of fiddling, lots of experimentation, and meanwhile the symptoms were coming and going."

For Peggy, the most troubling symptom was her "fuzzy thinking"; the lapses in concentration affected her job. Because so many of the women on the managerial level at her company are about her age, Peggy decided to start a support group at the office. She got nowhere fast. "Maybe I was naive about the stigma," she says. "These women didn't even want to talk to their husbands about menopause, much less their boss. They were reluctant to band together and accept the label *menopausal.* I wanted to invite in my doctor and do a seminar, but the other managers were scared the men would hold it against them, that they'd think 'Oh God, we've got a group of menopausal women running this company.'"

Incapable by her very nature of letting a good idea drop so easily, Peggy began leading discussions for other support groups, doing the program she'd designed for her own co-workers at other offices. The reluctance of her friends to come out of the closet still rankles her. "Professional women really need to talk to each other," she says. "They're so busy that they're closed off, but we have to have unity to demand the attention of the medical community and to dissolve the stigma at work.

"The joke is that menopausal women already are running this company, and a lot of other companies, and they're doing a fine job of it. But because these smart, competent women won't acknowledge the fact that they're in menopause, the old stereotypes about weepy, hysterical women roll right along."

The Rituals of Perimenopause

Our society provides no rite to mark the passage of perimenopause. We don't go into the woods to commune with nature, stand before an altar in a white dress, or throw each other un-baby showers. There are no dances, ceremonies, or chants to publicly announce that we've reached this particular milestone.

But some of the women with whom we spoke devised rituals of their own, personal ways to acknowledge that something in their lives had changed. Two women took trips. One went alone, to China, a place she always swore she would visit. The other three friends along with their adult daughters, retraced the grand tour that the older women had taken of Europe after their college graduation 40 years earlier. Now a framed picture of the seven women on the Spanish Steps hangs beside the circa-1954 picture of the older four as young girls, standing on the same steps in the same pose, laughing and squinting into the same blazing Italian sun.

Sometimes the rituals were not ones of closure but sprang from a desire to do something completely new. After menopause, some women felt a sudden zing of energy that prompted them to take up sports or hobbies, sign up for classes, audition for a play at the local theater, move to a new house. One woman changed the spelling of her name.

Perhaps the most elaborate ritual we came across was the slumber party that Peggy, the woman we met earlier, threw to celebrate her 50th birthday. "I definitely did plan this party to be symbolic," she says. "It was all about letting go and moving on to the next stage of life. I invited only women to come, although my new husband had a little problem with that. He wanted to know if he just couldn't stop by when we cut the cake, but I said that this party was to celebrate all the things women do when they're alone together. I was very selective, chose the best friends from all the different aspects of my life without worrying about whether or not everyone knew each other."

A friend who owned a vintage clothing store brought over all her finery, and after the women played dress-up and each chose a fancy hat, Peggy read aloud the valentines she'd written for her friends over the previous weeks. "I told each friend what was special about her and how important she'd been in my life as a woman. After I read them, everybody was crying, and they said, 'It's your birthday. We should have made valentines for you.'

"I'd anticipated that, so I took them into another room where I'd set out all sorts of craft stuff—construction paper, doilies, glitter and ribbons and glue—and I let them make valentines for me. That was a very important part of the ritual, the single biggest issue I've had to come to grips with lately. I used to try to do everything for everybody else, but in this stage of life I'm going to let other people do nice things for me."

As the evening wore on, the silliness accelerated. The women played relay races, passed LifeSavers on toothpicks, braided each other's hair, told ghost stories, watched movies late into the night on TV, and finally dozed in sleeping bags. The next morning they made pancakes for breakfast and went home. "It was one of the happiest days of my life," Peggy says. "The ritual worked. I don't complain about getting old anymore. . . . I keep the valentines in a big box, and I read them when I get down to remind myself how many friends I have, how loved I really am."

Afterword

We're not trying to suggest that if you follow every piece of advice in this book, life will be perfect or menopause will be easy. The best strategy is to get as much information as you can but approach the experience with an open mind. Women who are determined never to take HRT are rather like the women who enter childbirth vowing that they'll do it "naturally" no matter what. Don't set yourself up for disappointment. Menopause is different for everyone, problems may arise you couldn't foresee, and the important thing is to be well-informed about the alternatives. With any luck, you'll sail through menopause. But if it turns out to be tougher than you anticipated, seeking medical intervention doesn't make you a failure.

The good news is that the earlier you start preparing for menopause, the less likely you are to be thrown by it. Women don't need to have a physician's knowledge to be proactive in their own health care, but they do need to educate themselves about HRT and the effect diet, exercise, vitamin therapy, and stress reduction can have on their lives.

Throughout the 1990s, 4,000 women will enter menopause each day, and as our numbers grow, so does the strength of our voice. We have the right to expect that our complaints be taken seriously, that women's illnesses receive as much funding and research as men's, and that support systems exist to help us through perimenopause and beyond. We can and should fulfill many of these expectations for ourselves, but some require acknowledgment from the larger community.

The first step in getting what we need is to admit that we need it. As Peggy pointed out in the previous chapter, as long as we are reluctant to claim the word *menopausal,* we are accepting the stigma society has placed on the term and perpetuating the myths. We need to be vocal about our expectations, especially to our own doctors, and take heart from the fact that our very numbers guarantee we won't be ignored. While menopause may once have changed women, this generation has the opportunity to change menopause.

Sources

American Cancer Society
19 West 56th St.
New York, NY 10019
(212) 586-8700

The society offers information on giving up smoking.

American College of Ob Gyn
Office of Public Information
409 12th St. NW
Washington, DC 20024-2188
(202) 638-5577

This organization publishes newsletters, pamphlets, and a list of physicians specializing in childbirth and the diseases of women.

American Fertility Society
1209 Montgomery Hwy.
Birminghgam, AL 35216-2809
(205) 978-5000

Call or write for a listing of reproductive endocrinologists as well as information on perimenopausal fertility.

American Lung Association
1740 Broadway
New York, NY 10019
(212) 315-8700

The association offers information on giving up smoking.

American Sleep Disorders Association/
National Sleep Foundation
122 S. Robertson Blvd., Third Floor
Los Angeles, CA 90048
(310) 288-0466

General information and manuals on sleep hygiene are offered, as well as the locations and programs offered at sleep disorder clinics across the country.

Biofeedback Society of America
10200 West 44th Ave.
Wheat Ridge, CO 80033
(303) 422-8436

The society offers guidance on where to find a biofeedback center or a qualified practitioner as well as general information on the variety of physical disorders that can be improved through this technique.

Good Vibrations
1210 Valencia St.
San Francisco, CA 94110
(415) 974-8990

This San Francisco-based store is a well-known mail-order source of vibrators and other sexual aids.

National Alliance of Breast Cancer Organizations
1180 Avenue of the Americas
New York, NY 10036
(212) 719-0154

This is a clearinghouse for the many organizations offering information on prevention and treatment and the progress we're making (or not making) on breast cancer as a national health issue.

National Center for Homeopathy
810 North Fairfax, Suite 306
Alexandria, VA 22314
(703) 548-7790

The center sponsors conferences, publishes a newsletter, and sells books. Its Directory of Homeopathic Practitioners ($5) is your best source for a qualified local homeopath.

National Osteoporosis Foundation
1150 17th St. NW, Suite 500
Washington, DC 20036
(202) 223-2226

The National Osteoporosis Foundation offers information on calcium, exercise, diagnostic procedures such as DEXA, and the latest research on how to prevent and reverse bone loss.

North American Menopause Society
University Hospitals Department of Ob Gyn
2074 Abington Rd.
Cleveland, OH 44106
(212) 844-3334

The NAMS can refer you to a local physician with specialized training in menopause and also has a recommended reading list.

Further Reading

Estrogen: Yes or No? Morris Notelovitz, M.D., Ph.D. and Diana Tonnessen, St. Martin's Press. Facts on hormone replacement therapy, with the pros and cons outlined, excerpted from *Menopause and Midlife Health.* Short and to the point.

Menopause and Midlife Health Morris Notelovitz, M.D., Ph.D., and Diana Tonnessen, St. Martin's Press. Encyclopedic reference book on women's health by one of the leaders in the field. If you have a question, the answer can probably be found here.

Hormones, Hot Flashes and Mood Swings Clark Gillespie, M.D., Harper Perennial. Full of factoids about perimenopause, menopause, and postmenopause. The format tends to break up the continuity of thought. The chapter on "The Menopause and the Bedroom" is so silly it borders on offensive.

Estrogen Lila E. Nachtigall, M.D., and Joan Rattner Heilman, Harper Perennial. The title is misleading because this is really a good basic book about menopause, its symptoms, and its health consequences. Estrogen figures in the discussion as a treatment, but is certainly not the book's sole focus. Dr. Nachtigall is one of the most experienced physicians in the field and offers practical advice.

The Pause Lonnie Barbach, Ph.D., Dutton (Penguin Books). Personal and anecdotal information on menopause. The chapter on alternative therapies (homeopathy, acupuncture, herbs) is an unusual addition to an otherwise basic discussion of menopause.

Managing Your Menopause Wulf H. Utian, M.D., Ph.D., and Ruth S. Jacobowitz, Simon and Schuster. A leading expert offers his personal and very directive advice.

Stop the Insanity! Susan Powter, Simon and Schuster. Entertaining personal account of how Ms. Powter took control of her eating, exercise, and sanity, and how you can do the same. Underneath the hype is some good, practical advice.

Menopause Self Help Book Susan M. Lark, M.D., Celestial-Arts. Highlights a nonhormonal approach to menopause, using nutritional supplements, exercise programs, and stress-reduction techniques. Information on symptoms and health risks is bare bones, however, and many women will need more information than what's offered before making the HRT versus no-HRT decision.

The Silent Passage: Menopause Gail Sheehy, Random House. A ground-breaking work on the social and psychological aspects of menopause combined with solid, broad-based medical information. Still the champ!

Stay Cool through Menopause Melvin Frisch, M.D., The Body Press/Perigee Books. A question-and-answer format, focusing on the medical aspects of menopause, with very little information on the psychological and emotional issues.

A Woman Doctor's Guide to Menopause Lois Jovanovic, M.D., with Suzanne Levert, Hyperion. Matter-of-fact discussion of all the medical concerns of menopause. Less attention paid to the larger quality-of-life issues and the importance of menopause as a gateway to the future.

Menopause and the Years Ahead Mary Beard, M.D., and Lindsay Curtis, M.D., Fisher Books. A question-and-answer approach, with some fairly clinical illustrations. Covers a few areas, such as cosmetic surgery and aging issues, that other books only skim.

Making Sense of Menopause Faye Kitchener Cone, Simon and Schuster. Excellent overview intermingled with comments from mid-life women discussing their personal experiences. Written in a conversational tone, easy to understand.

Rationalizations for Women Who Do Too Much While Running with the Wolves Allison McCune and Tomye B. Spears, Bob Adams, Inc. This book offers rationalizations for everything from not recycling to not having sex, saving the busy woman from having to stop and think of her own excuses. Laughter *is* the best medicine.

Glossary

Abortion: pregnancy loss, usually by 20 weeks gestation, either spontaneous (naturally occurring) or induced (medically or surgically).

Aerobic exercise: activities requiring oxygen for prolonged periods, improving the body's capacity to handle oxygen.

Amenorrhea: absence of menstrual periods.

Androgens: hormones that produce male or masculine characteristics.

Artificial insemination: placement of sperm into the female reproductive tract by means other than sexual intercourse.

Basal body temperature (BBT): temperature taken immediately upon awakening before any activity; this temperature rises coincident with a rise in progesterone level, as occurs following ovulation. Can be used to determine approximate time of ovulation, either to attempt or avoid pregnancy.

Calcium: mineral essential to building strong bones and teeth.

DEXA: dual energy X ray absorptiometry, a low-dose X ray technique for measuring bone density.

Endometriosis: disease where tissue from the lining of the uterus grows in areas outside the uterus; thought to originate when menstrual blood flows backward out the fallopian tubes into the pelvic cavity.

Endometrium: hormonally responsive lining of the uterine cavity, shed every (nonpregnant) cycle as menstruation.

Estradiol: primary and most potent estrogen produced by the ovaries.

Estrogen: female hormone produced by the ovaries during reproductive years, responsible for female sexual characteristics.

Estrone: a weak estrogen derived from estradiol.

Fallopian tube: tube extending from the ovary to the uterus that acts as conduit for sperm to the egg.

Fecundity: the ability to achieve pregnancy (resulting in a live birth) within one menstrual cycle.

Fertility: the ability to conceive and bear a child.

Follicle: saclike structure within the ovary containing an egg.

Follicle-stimulating hormone (FSH):   pituitary hormone that stimulates the ovary to mature follicles for ovulation; associated with increasing estrogen production throughout the menstrual cycle. An elevated FSH level is a sign of menopause.

Formication: tingling sensation, as though insects are crawling on the skin; rare symptom associated with menopause.

GIFT (gamete intra-fallopian transfer): infertility treatment in which eggs and sperm are mixed together and placed into a woman's fallopian tube, usually via laparoscopy.

HDL cholesterol: smallest and most dense of the substances that transport fats in the blood. High levels of HDL are protective against cardiovascular disease.

Hormone: chemical messenger produced by a special tissue; it is released into the blood and then travels to distant cells where it exerts its specific effect.

HRT (hormone replacement therapy): use of estrogen and progesterone to supply the body with hormones that the ovary no longer makes after menopause.

Hysterectomy: surgical removal of the uterus. A "complete" hysterectomy refers to the removal of the tubes and ovaries along with the uterus.

Infertility: one year of unprotected intercourse without conception.

In vitro fertilization: fertilization of an egg by sperm in a laboratory dish or test tube with placement of the resultant embryo into the woman's uterus.

Kegel exercises: contracting the muscles around the urethra, bladder, and rectum to improve control of urination.

Laparoscopy: surgical procedure using long, thin telescope inserted through the umbilicus to view the internal pelvic/reproductive organs.

LDL cholesterol: low-density lipoprotein carrying cholesterol to blood vessel walls, associated with increased risk of coronary disease.

Libido: sex drive.

Luteal phase: portion of the menstrual cycle from ovulation to the onset of the next menstrual period.

Luteinizing hormone (LH):   pituitary hormone that stimulates progesterone production by the ovary and triggers release of the egg.

Mammogram: X ray of the breast to screen for cancer.

Menarche: occurrence of first menstrual period.

Menopause: cessation of menstruation due to depletion of ovarian follicles (eggs), the end of a woman's ability to reproduce.

Menstrual cycle: a woman's monthly reproductive cycle, with stimulation of ovarian follicular growth and ovulation, corresponding hormone production and resultant thickening of the uterine lining, and shedding of this lining as a menstrual period if pregnancy does not occur.

Oophorectomy: surgical removal of the ovaries.

Osteoporosis: thinning of bone from loss of calcium.

Ovarian failure: inability of the ovary to produce estrogen and progesterone, loss of follicles containing eggs; menopause.

Ovary: organ in the female containing eggs and producing sex hormones.

Ovulation: release of an egg from the ovary.

Perimenopause: transition years leading up to the last menstrual period or menopause.

PMS (premenstrual syndrome):   physical and psychological/emotional symptoms associated with the postovulatory (luteal) phase of the menstrual cycle. Usually followed by a time entirely free of symptoms.

Progesterone: hormone produced by the ovary after ovulation.

Progestin: synthetic hormone with progesterone-like effects; used along with estrogen in HRT.

Reproductive endocrinology: study of the hormonal regulation of reproduction and the menstrual cycle.

Stress incontinence: loss of urine with cough or sneeze.

Tamoxifen: drug that acts as anti-estrogen, countering the effects of estrogen and used in the prevention and treatment of breast cancer.

Testosterone: male hormone produced by the testes in men and, in small amounts, by the ovary in women.

Transdermal: through the skin.

Uterus: female organ in which the fetus develops and is carried throughout a pregnancy. The opening of the uterus in the vagina is the cervix.

Vagina: birth canal, leading from the uterus/cervix to the outside of a woman's body.

Vaginal atrophy: thinning of the vaginal walls due to lack of estrogen.

Weight-bearing exercise: physical activity requiring participants to use their extremities to carry their full weight. Walking and jogging are weight-bearing exercises; swimming is not.

Weight-resistance exercise: exercise requiring contraction of a muscle and then movement of a joint or extremity against a weight or force (such as a resistance band).

ZIFT (zygote intra-fallopian transfer): infertility treatment involving placement of an in vitro fertilized egg into a woman's fallopian tube.

Zygote: egg that has been penetrated (fertilized) by a sperm.

Index